BASIC GUIDE TO INFECTION PREVENTION AND CONTROL IN DENTISTRY

Caroline L. Pankhurst and Wilson A. Coulter

WILEY-BLACKWELL

A John Wiley & Sons, Ltd., Publication

Blackwell Publishing was acquired by John Wiley & Sons in February 2007.
Blackwell's publishing programme has been merged with Wiley's global Scientific, Technical,
and Medical business to form Wiley-Blackwell.

Registered office
John Wiley & Sons Ltd., The Atrium, Southern Gate, Chichester, West Sussex, PO19 8SQ,
United Kingdom

Editorial offices
9600 Garsington Road, Oxford, OX4 2DQ, United Kingdom
2121 State Avenue, Ames, Iowa 50014-8300, USA

For details of our global editorial offices, for customer services and for information about how to
apply for permission to reuse the copyright material in this book please see our website at
www.wiley.com/wiley-blackwell.

Library of Congress Cataloging-in-Publication Data
Pankhurst, Caroline.
Basic guide to infection prevention and control in dentistry / Caroline L. Pankhurst
and Wilson A. Coulter.
p. ; cm.
Includes bibliographical references and index.
ISBN 978-1-4051-7662-0 (pbk. : alk. paper)   1. Dental offices—Sanitation.
2. Cross infection—Prevention.   3. Dentistry—Safety measures.
4. Mouth—Infection—Prevention.   I. Coulter, Wilson.   II. Title.
[DNLM: 1. Dental Health Services—organization & administration.   2. Infection Control,
Dental.   3. Cross Infection—prevention & control.   4. Risk Management.
WU 29 P193b 2009]

RK52.P36 2009
617.6—dc22

2008047430

A catalogue record for this book is available from the British Library.

Set in 10/12.5 pt Sabon by Aptara® Inc., New Delhi, India
Printed in Singapore

1   2009

Contents

Chapter 1
Essentials of infection control

WHY DO WE NEED INFECTION CONTROL IN DENTISTRY?

WHY DO WE NEED INFECTION CONTROL IN DENTISTRY?

Dentists are exposed to a wide variety of potentially infectious microorganisms in their clinical environment. The transmission of infectious agents from person to person or from inanimate objects within the clinical environment resulting in infection is known as *cross-infection*.

The protocols and procedures involved in the prevention and control of infection in dentistry are directed to reduce the possibility or *risk* of cross-infection occurring in the dental clinic, thereby producing a safe environment for both patients and staff.

All employers have a legal obligation under the Health and Safety at Work Act 1974 to ensure that all their employees are appropriately trained and proficient in the procedures necessary for working safely. They are also required by the *Control of Substances Hazardous to Health* (COSHH) *Regulations 2002* to review every procedure carried out by their employees which involves contact with a substance hazardous to health, including pathogenic microorganisms. Employers and their employees are also responsible in law to ensure that any person on the premises, including patients, contractors and visitors, is not placed at any *avoidable risk*, as far as is reasonably practicable.

Thus, the concept of the risk of cross-infection is an important one in dentistry. We do not deal in absolutes, but our infection control measures are directed towards reducing, to an acceptable level, the probability or possibility that an infection could be transmitted. This is usually measured against the background infection rate expected in the local population; i.e. the patient or dental operative system is placed at no increased risk of infection when entering the dental environment. Infection control guidance in dental surgery has developed from an assessment of the evidence base, consideration of the best clinical practice and risk assessment (Figure 1.1).

How we manage the prevention of cross-infection and control the risk of spread of infection in the dental clinic is the subject of this book.

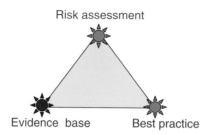

Figure 1.1 The basis of the development of infection control guidance in dental surgery.

RELATIVE RISK AND RISK PERCEPTION

Risk has many definitions and is perceived by the dental profession and the public in different ways which can have an impact on the perception of the public and dental staff as to how safe it is in the dental clinic. For example, risks which are under personal control, such as driving a car, are more acceptable than the risks of travelling by aeroplane or train. Thus, the public often perceives travelling by car to be safer than by air even though the accident statistics do not support this perception. Unseen risks such as infection and particularly those with frightening consequences such as AIDS or MRSA are predictably most alarming to the profession and the public. Risks can be clinical, environmental, financial, economic or political, as well as those affecting public perception and reputation of the dentist.

What makes risks significant? There are a number of criteria which make risks significant and worthy of concern:

- Potential for actual injury to patients or staff

- Significant occupational health and safety hazard

- The possibility of erosion of reputation or public confidence

- Potential for litigation

- Minor incidents which occur in clusters and may represent trends

Understanding what is implied by the term *hazard* is important when we consider the control of infection. This may be defined as a situation, or substance, including microorganisms, with the potential to cause harm. Thus, risk must take into account not only the likelihood or probability that a particular hazard may impact on the patient or dental staff but the severity of the consequences if it did impact on people.

RISK ASSESSMENT AND THE MANAGEMENT DECISION-MAKING PROCESS

It is the role of managers of dental practices to manage risk. The Management of Health and Safety at Work Regulations 1999 requires employers to carry out a risk assessment as an essential part of a risk management strategy. Infection control is an application of risk management to the dental clinical setting.

> *Risk management involves identification, assessment and analysis of risks and the implementation of risk control procedures designed to eliminate or reduce the risk.*

Risk control in dentistry is a single-tier approach in which all patients are treated without discrimination as though they were potentially infectious. This approach was previously referred to as *universal precautions* and has been replaced by *standard precautions* which treat all body fluids, with the exception of sweat, as a source of infection and include a series of measures and procedures designed to prevent exposure of staff or patients to direct contact with infected body fluids. Specifically, dental health care workers (HCWs) should provide barriers to exchange of blood, saliva and gingival fluid between operator and patient and patient and operator.

Decisions made within an organisation, and within practice, should take into account the potential risks that could directly or indirectly affect a patient's care. If risks are properly assessed, the process can help all health care professionals and organisations set their priorities and improve decision-making to reach an optimal balance of risk, benefit and cost. If dental teams systematically identify, assess, learn from and manage all risks and incidents, they will be able to reduce potential and actual risks, and identify opportunities to improve health care.

Risk assessment has the following benefits for delivery of dental health care:

- Strives for the optimal balance of risk by focusing on the reduction or mitigation of risk while supporting and fostering innovation, so that greatest returns can be achieved with acceptable results, costs and risks

- Supports better decision-making through a solid understanding of all risks and their likely impact

- Enables dentist to plan for uncertainty, with well-considered contingency plans which cope with the impact of unexpected events and increase staff, patient and public confidence in care that is delivered

- Helps the dentist comply with published standards and guidelines

- Highlights weakness and vulnerability in procedures, practices and policy changes

HOW TO PERFORM A RISK ASSESSMENT IN A DENTAL PRACTICE

A risk assessment in dental practice involves five stages:

1. Look for the hazards

2. Decide who might be harmed, and how

3. Evaluate the risks arising from the hazards and decide whether existing precautions are adequate or should more be done

4. Record your findings

5. Review your assessment periodically and revise it if necessary

Stage 1: Look for the hazards

- Divide your work into manageable categories

- Concentrate on significant hazards, which could result in serious harm or affect several people

- Ask your employees for their views; involve the whole dental team

- Separate activities into operational stages to ensure that there are no hidden hazards

- Make use of manufacturers' datasheets to help you spot hazards and put risks in their true perspective

- Review past accidents and ill-health records

Stage 2: Who might be harmed?

- Identify all members of staff at risk from the significant hazard

- Do not forget people who only come into contact with the hazard infrequently, e.g. maintenance contractors, visitors, general public and people sharing your workplace

- Highlight those persons particularly at risk who may be more vulnerable, e.g. the young, people with disabilities, inexperienced or temporary workers and lone workers

Stage 3: Evaluate the level of risk

- The aim is to reduce all risks to a low level
- Determine for each significant hazard if the remaining risk, after all precautions have been taken, is *high*, *medium* or *low*
- Concentrate on the greatest risks first
- Examine how work is actually carried out and identify failures to follow procedures or practices
- Need to comply with legal requirements and standards
- The law says that you must do what is reasonably practical to keep your workplace safe

A numerical evaluation of risk can be made to help prioritise the need for action and allow comparison of relative risk. *Risk* is equal to *severity* multiplied by *likelihood*. Assign a score of 1–5 for each, with a total value of 16–25 equating to *high risk*, 9–15 to *medium risk* and >8 to *low risk* (Figure 1.2).

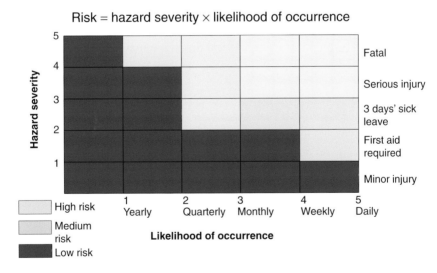

Figure 1.2 Graph showing how hazard severity and likelihood of occurrence are related to risk.

Stage 4: Record your findings

Record the significant findings of your assessment and include significant hazards and important conclusions.

ESSENTIALS OF INFECTION CONTROL

Information to be recorded:

- Activities or work areas examined
- Hazards identified
- Persons exposed to the hazards
- Evaluation of risks and their prioritisation
- Existing control measures and their effectiveness
- What additional precautions are needed and who is to take action and when

Stage 5: Review your assessment

Risk assessment is a continuing process and must be kept up to date to ensure that it takes into account new activities and hazards, changes in processes, methods of work and new employees.

You must document your findings but there is no need to show how you did your assessment, provided you can show that a proper check was made and you *asked who* might be affected, and that you dealt with all the obvious significant hazards taking into account the *number of people* who could be involved, that the precautions taken are reasonable, and that the remaining risk is low.

HIERARCHY OF RISK MANAGEMENT CONTROL

Following a risk assessment is necessary to implement a plan to control the observed risk. The plan of action must set out in priority order what *additional controls are necessary*, and aim to reduce risks to an acceptable level and comply with relevant legal requirements. You must also establish a reasonable time scale for completion and decide who is responsible for taking the necessary action.

There is a hierarchy of control options which can be summarised as:

- Elimination (buy in services/goods)
- Substitution (use something less hazardous/risky)
- Enclosure (enclose to eliminate/control risks)
- Guarding/segregation (people/machines)
- Safe systems of work (reduce system to an acceptable level)
- Written procedures that are known and understood by those affected

- Adequate supervision

- Identification of training needs and implementation

- Information/instruction (signs, handouts, policies)

- Personal protective equipment (PPE)

These control measures can be applied as judged appropriate following the risk assessment, taking into account the legal requirements and standards, affordability and the views of the dental team.

INFECTION CONTROL AND THE LAW

Laws relating to infection control can arise from legal acts and orders from the individual county or as European Union Directives. A distinction must be made between *regulations* and *approved codes of practice* and *advice*.

Regulations are laws, approved by the national legislative body. In the UK, regulations that govern infection control come under the *Health Act 2006* and the *Health and Safety at Work Act*. This applies to regulations based on EC Directives as well as national regulations. The Health and Safety at Work Act and general duties in the management regulations are goal setting and give employers the freedom to decide how to control risks which they identify. However, some risks are so great or the proper control measures so costly that it would not be appropriate to leave the discretion on the employer to decide what to do about them. Regulations identify these risks and set out specific actions that must be taken. Often these requirements are absolute – to do something without qualification by deciding whether it is reasonably practicable.

Approved codes of practice (ACP) offer practical examples of good practice. They give advice on how to comply with the law by, for example, providing a guide to what is 'reasonably practicable'. For example, if regulations use words like 'suitable and sufficient', an ACP can illustrate what this requires in particular circumstances. ACP have a special *legal status*. If employers are prosecuted for a breach of health and safety law, and it is proved that they have not followed the relevant provisions of the ACP, court can find them at fault unless they show that they have complied with the law in some other way. The 'hygiene code', the full title being the Code of Practice for the Prevention and Control of Health Care Associated Infections (HCAIs), is an example of an ACP which was published under the *Health Act 2006* legislation. This code sets out criteria according to which managers of 'NHS organisations' are to ensure that patients are cared for in a clean environment where the risk of HCAI is as low as possible. In this context, a dental practice is an example of an NHS organisation, and must seek to comply with the ACP. If it fails to comply, then enforcement notices can be served to make improvement mandatory. Examples of a duty set out in this ACP, which is guided by the recommendations outlined in Chapters 5 and 7, include:

- Adequate provision of suitable hand-washing facilities and antibacterial hand rubs
- There are effective arrangements for the appropriate decontamination of instruments and other equipment

This ACP also emphasises that NHS bodies must comply with all relevant legislation such as the Health and Safety at Work Act 1974 and COSHH regulations.

LEGAL ACTS UNDER WHICH DENTAL PRACTICE IS CONDUCTED

The Health Act 2006

The Health Act 2006 is the latest update of health legislation which is applied in the UK. This lays out the framework for the provision of health care and the responsibilities of the various bodies and professionals tasked with the delivery of health care including dentists. (Further information can be found at http://www.dh.gov.uk/en/Publicationsandstatistics/Legislation/Actsandbills/DH_064103.)

The Health and Safety at Work Act 1974

Employers have a duty under the law to ensure, 'so far as is reasonably practicable', the health, safety and welfare of their staff and members of the public at their place of work. This legislation is periodically updated and the *Management of Health and Safety at Work Regulations 1999* made more explicit what employers are required to do to manage health and safety. In particular, this act required employers to look at what the risks are in their workplace and take sensible measures to tackle, i.e. to carry out risk assessments as discussed above. It is the duty of the employer to *consult with staff* on matters which may impact on their health and safety at work including:

- Any change which may substantially affect their health and safety at work, e.g. in procedures, equipment or ways of working

- The employer's arrangements for getting competent people to help him/her satisfy health and safety laws

- The information you have to be given on the likely risks and dangers arising from your work, measures to reduce or get rid of these risks and what you should do if you have to deal with a risk or danger

- The planning of health and safety

- The health and safety consequences of introducing new technology

The duties of employers under this law include:

- Making your workplace safe and without risks to health

- Ensuring plant and machinery are safe and that safe systems of work are set and followed

- Ensuring articles and substances are moved, stored and used safely

- Providing adequate welfare facilities

- Giving the information, instruction, training and supervision necessary for the heath and safety of staff and the public (http://www.hse.gov.uk/pubns/law.pdf)

Control of Substances Hazardous to Health Regulations 2002

The law requires employers to control exposure to hazardous substances to prevent ill health. They have to protect both employees and others who may be exposed by complying with the COSHH regulations. COSHH is a useful tool of good management which sets basic measures, with a simple step-by-step approach, that employers, and sometimes employees, must take which will help to assess risks, implement any measures needed to control exposure and establish good working practices.

> Note that hazardous substances include not only chemicals such as mercury, solvents and the materials used in dentistry, but also biological agents such as bacteria and other microorganisms.

The regulations require risk assessment to be made on all the materials used in dental practice and further information can be found on the web at http://www.hse.gov.uk/pubns/indg136.pdf.

ESSENTIALS OF INFECTION CONTROL

The Reporting of Injuries, Diseases and Dangerous Occurrences 1995

Reporting accidents and ill health at work is a legal requirement. The information enables the health and safety executive (HSE) and local authorities to identify where and how risks arise and to investigate serious accidents. As an employer, a person who is self-employed, or someone in control of work premises, you have legal duties under the Reporting of Injuries, Diseases and Dangerous Occurrences (RIDDOR) 1995 that require you to report and record some work-related accidents by the quickest means possible. You must report deaths, major injuries and an injury which results in the employee or self-employed person being away from work or unable to perform their normal work duties for more than three consecutive days. Thus, the dental surgery must be an environment where we positively encourage accident reporting by all of the dental team. (Further information on reporting accidents can be found at http://www.hse.gov.uk/riddor/index.htm.)

The Pressure Systems Safety Regulations 2000

Because autoclaves are pressurised vessels and are potentially explosive, they come under legal requirements to be tested annually to ensure safety and also for insurance purposes. The Pressure Systems Safety Regulations came into force in 2000. Users and owners of pressure systems are required to demonstrate that they know the safe operating limits, principally pressure and temperature, of their pressure systems and that the systems are safe under those conditions. They need to ensure that a suitable written scheme of examination is in place before the system is operated. They also need to ensure that the pressure system is actually examined in accordance with the written scheme of examination. These safety tests are also required for insurance purposes (http://www.hse.gov.uk/pubns/indg178.pdf).

PUBLISHED STANDARDS AND GUIDANCE

Standards and guidance relating to infection control are set and can be obtained from a number of sources such as:

- *Health and Safety Executive* is a regulatory body with the responsibility to promote better health and safety at work, provide an information and advisory service, and submit proposals for new or revised regulations and approved codes of practice (www.hse.gov.uk)

- *Medicine and Health Products Regulatory Agency* (formerly Medical Devices Agency) ensures that medicines and medical devices work and are acceptably safe (http://www.mhra.gov.uk)

- *The National Institute for Health and Clinical Excellence* (NICE) is an independent organisation responsible for providing national guidance on the promotion of good health and the prevention and treatment of ill health specifically for HCWs as well as guidance on the use of new and existing medicines, treatments and procedures within the health service (http://www.nice.org.uk/)

- *Department of Environment, Food and Rural Affairs* gives advice on chemicals and waste disposal, which is discussed in Chapter 10 (http://www.defra.gov.uk/Environment/index.htm)

- *British Dental Association* provides advice on infection control through their infection control advisory sheets for members, which have been a useful source of guidance to dentist in the UK (http://www.bda.org/)

- *General Dental Council* (GDC) is a professional organisation which regulates dental professionals in the UK and maintains standards in dental practice in the interest of patients by emphasising training and competence. The GDC, for example, has advised dentists to:

  - 'Find out about laws and regulations which affect your work, premises, equipment and business, and follow them'

  - 'Provide a good standard of care based on available up-to-date evidence and reliable guidance' (http://www.gdc-uk.org/)

Policy

The arms of government, outlined above, dictate policy which is published in the form of strategic documents which they seek to implement. These policies are often the result of special advisory bodies such as the Spongiform Encephalopathy Advisory Committee (SEAC; http://www.seac.gov.uk/).

When the Department of Health agrees on a strategy, it cascades this down to those local organisations which are tasked with implementation such as a local health authority. Health service circulars and letters of the chief dental officer are used to communicate with the people in the dental profession and these can be accessed on the websites of your local area.

Procedures

Recommendations on procedures which are undertaken in dental practice are in the forms of device bulletins, health technical memorandum (HTM) and model engineering specifications, which provide essential information if we are to keep up to date with what would be considered good practice.

Device bulletins

Device bulletins are produced by the Department of Health and contain guidance and information on medical devices of a more general management interest. They are written as a result of experience gained from adverse incident investigations, contacts with manufacturers and users, and device evaluations. Bulletins are often written in response to adverse incidence where there is a need to communicate changes in practice following from the experience gained when an incident has occurred (http://www.mhra. gov.uk/Publications/Safetyguidance/DeviceBulletins/index.htm).

Health technical memorandum

These publications give advice and guidance on specific health care topics and set out recommendations for good practice. An example of an HTM is HTM 01-01, the first part of the Decontamination Series, which has a major impact on dental practice in the UK. This HTM provides guidance on choice, specification, purchase, installation, validation, periodic testing, operation and maintenance of the sterilisers. The dental profession has been working towards implementing the recommendations of this HTM and that of the more recently published HTM 01-05, and the practices and procedures covered in Chapter 7 are based largely on these recommendations.

Model engineering specifications

Model engineering specifications give detailed information on equipment, its use and maintenance, etc., and are used as a source of reference by engineers who the dentists will have to employ to test and validate, for example, the autoclaves and thermal washer-disinfectors used in dental practice, which are discussed in Chapter 7.

Implementation

The implementation of policy and procedures has to be monitored at the local level and this has been incorporated into *quality assurance* and *clinical governance*. *Clinical governance* has been introduced as a new approach to quality improvement in the NHS within the UK, with the aim of measuring and improving quality of care. Governance incorporates existing activities such as clinical audit, education and training, research and development, and risk management. Thus, many of the activities related to infection control and prevention are monitored and assessed when applying clinical governance to the dental practice. Clinical audit is a useful tool which can be very effectively applied to infection control, and indeed making a comparison of our activities against the standards outlined in the sources discussed above is required when conducting an audit, which is an integral part of our practice to improve standards of care and safety.

Further information on clinical governance and its relationship with clinical and managerial approaches to the quality of care can be found in a paper by Buetow and Roland (1999; http://qshc.bmj.com/cgi/reprint/8/3/184).

TEAM APPROACH TO PREVENTION OF INFECTION

It is now accepted that a team approach is required in dentistry to improve the care which we deliver to our patients. The advantage of teamwork is that teams would:

- Utilise the skill mix within the profession by using the talents of the whole dental team
- Allow the whole dental team, not just dentists, to give their best to NHS dentistry
- Help to improve quality and cost-effectiveness

The emphasis on developing dental teams by the GDC has resulted in the publication of *Developing the Dental Team* (2004) and a new register for professions complementary to dentistry (PCD) to include dental nurses, technicians, clinical dental technicians, orthodontic therapists as well as dental hygienists and therapists.

A team is more than just a group of people working together; it has been defined as:

A small number of people with complementary skills who are committed to a common purpose, performance goals and approach for which they hold themselves mutually accountable.

Infection control of necessity requires a team approach and each member of the team must have complementary skills and share the common purpose to ensure safe practice. 'For the team to function effectively there must be clear goals shared by the team, good communication between the team members, with clear, fair leadership and an open climate based on respect and absence of a blame culture'. This will encourage staff to feel confident and safe to treat patients with potentially infectious disease and express their concerns on infection matters and thus contribute to the improvement of service delivery. Generally, teamwork improves job satisfaction, increases the sense of being valued and encourages a collective responsibility for the delivery of service.

Effective leadership is an important constituent of the dental team and they must provide a clear vision of the standard of excellence which the team is seeking to achieve and communicate this to the members of the team. This is best achieved by ensuring that there is adequate training for dental nurses (dental care professionals (DCPs)), hygienist, receptionists, etc., in infection control and that there are regular clinical management meetings within the practice. Meetings are required to allow communication between the team members and for risk assessments to be made as new problems arise. There is evidence that busy dental practices do not have regular structured team meeting built into their routine, and particularly in the rapidly developing field of infection control these meetings are essential.

Communication is essential if the members of the dental team are to report accidents and feedback their opinions, reservations and fears regarding infection control policy and conditions of work in the dental practice. Individuals must not be discouraged by the perception of 'failure' if they report accidents or incidents.

It is useful to consider what the causes of human failure are, as human error is one of the greatest reasons for breaches in infection control practice. Failure is usually caused by either:

- *Errors in knowledge* where the HCWs did not know what they were suppose to do to, for example, the importance of safe disposal of sharps and the prevention of transmission of infection by aerosol in the clinic

- *Errors in skills* where the HCWs did not have sufficient training to, for example, carry out procedures such as decontaminate an instrument or use a scalpel safely

There may be an environment in the dental surgery which due to poor organisation and failure in management is conducive to personal failure and errors. The reduction of human error is therefore closely related to good practice management and to having an effective team.

Human error can be minimised by improving job design, i.e. ensuring that everyone knows his or her duties and has the skills to accomplish the tasks; preventing boredom by job rotation and job enrichment; and multi-skilling – which gives the HCW new challenges and maintains interest and pride in 'a job well done'.

Lastly, encouraging staff participation in decision-making and making them a valued member of the dental health care team will reduce errors, and if they occur they will be quickly corrected and be unlikely to reoccur.

REFERENCES AND WEBSITES

The Health Act 2006: Available at http://www.dh.gov.uk/en/Publicationsandstatistics/ Legislation/Actsandbills/DH_064103.

The Health and Safety at Work Act 1974: Available at http://www.hse.gov.uk/pubns/ law.pdf.

COSHH 2002: Available at http://www.hse.gov.uk/pubns/indg136.pdf.

RIDDOR 1995: Available at http://www.hse.gov.uk/riddor/index.htm.

Pressure Systems Safety Regulations 2000: Available at http://www.hse.gov.uk/ pubns/indg178.pdf.

Buetow, S.A. and Roland, M. (1999). Clinical governance: Bridging the gap between managerial and clinical approaches to quality of care. *Quality of Health Care*, 8, 184–190. Available at http://qshc.bmj.com/cgi/reprint/8/3/184.

Device Bulletins: Available at http://www.mhra.gov.uk/Publications/Safetyguidance/ DeviceBulletins/index.htm.

General Dental Council (2004). *Developing the Dental Team: Curricula Frameworks for Registrable Qualifications for PCTs*. Available at http://www.gdc-uk.org/ News+publications+and+events/Publications/Guidance+documents/Developing+the +Dental+Team.htm.

Chapter 2

Communicable diseases in the dental surgery

HOW INFECTIONS ARE SPREAD

Microorganisms must attach to or penetrate the surfaces of the body in order to establish themselves, and they have the potential to cause infection and disease in the host. This association between microbes and human cells is very specific and has evolved over millions of years; thus, many species of bacteria which colonise the mouth and oral tissues are not found anywhere else in the human body or at any other site in the biosphere.

While the body is well protected by intact skin, the orifices of the body are sites of potential entry for infection and are protected by secretions such as saliva and tears and defence mechanisms such as tonsils and lymph nodes. However, they remain a potential weak link in our defences, and hence we wear protective clothing such as masks to protect the respiratory tree, lips and mouth from infection and goggles to protect the eyes as part of infection control and prevention protocols.

The vast majority of microbes do not cause infection in humans; indeed a *resident* or *commensal* flora on the skin or in the gut and mouth is essential for health. These bacteria live in harmony with our body and protect us by preventing other more harmful bacteria attaching to and colonising the body. An example of this is seen in dental plaque where the species such as *Streptococcus sanguis* is associated with health and *Streptococcus mutans* with rampant caries in patients on high-sucrose diets.

Some microbes which are considered commensal and harmless can cause infection and disease when the host's immune system is compromised by, for example, age, diseases such as diabetes or cystic fibrosis, or infection such as human immunodeficiency virus (HIV). These are called *opportunist pathogens* and for this reason dentist must take particular care in taking a medical history of patients to enquire about conditions which may make patients more susceptible to infection and take steps to protect these vulnerable patients.

A successful microorganism which can cause disease (*pathogen*) must have a means of transmission from host to host; otherwise it would eventually disappear. Some microbes such as avian influenza virus, rabies virus, variant Creutzfeldt–Jakob disease (vCJD) and *Salmonella* use animals as their main host and occasionally spread to humans. These are known as *zoonosis* and although are important in the food industry and agriculture, they do not usually pose a risk of infection in the dental clinic. Insects such as mosquitoes can act as a means of transmission of infection of malaria, and these infections may impact on dentistry as they are usually blood-borne infections and could be potentially transmitted during operative dentistry. The dental clinic offers the potential to transmit infection from person to person and the method of prevention of this transmission is the essence of cross-infection control.

RESERVOIRS AND SOURCES OF INFECTION

For infection to spread there must also be a source of infection, which is most often a patient attending for dental treatment, and these sources may present three stages of infection/colonisation:

- Patients suffering from an infectious disease known as the index case, e.g. influenza, measles, AIDS and tuberculosis (TB)

- Patients in the prodromal or convalescent stage of infection, e.g. herpes simplex virus (HSV) and varicella zoster virus (VZV)

- Healthy carriers of disease, e.g. *Streptococcus pyogenes* (sore throat), methicillin-resistant *Staphylococcus aureus* (MRSA), *Neisseria meningitidis* (meningitis) and *Haemophilus influenzae* (bronchitis)

Patients with acute infection are usually very infectious and release large numbers of microbes into the environment. Those with serious infections rarely attend for routine clinical dentistry, but the dentist must be able and willing to treat such people in a manner which will ensure the safety of other staff and patients and consistent with offering high standards of dental care to the patient. It is a good policy to postpone elective treatment during the infective period which improves the patient's comfort and eliminates the risk of infection.

Much attention has been focused on convalescent and asymptomatic carriers of infection as these patients are often infective and the infections represent some of the most serious risks of transmission in the dental practice and the carriers cannot be readily identified. Those patients who carry hepatitis B virus (HBV) and hepatitis C virus (HCV) cannot be identified, but a good medical history is useful since some people will know their carrier status.

Healthcare associated infection (HCAI) or hospital-acquired infection, or nosocomial infection are infections caught or emerge while in hospital, for instance, infections caught from other patients or during treatment, and are a major cause of concern to the medical profession. Infections are considered

HAI if they first appear 48 hours or more after hospital admission or within 30 days after discharge from hospital. Prevalence rates vary greatly but are of the order of 10% in many countries, with urinary tract infection and pneumonia being most prevalent. Outbreaks of MRSA, *Clostridium difficile* and antibiotic multi-resistant organisms have created much anxiety amongst patients and the dental team must know how to prevent the spread of these microbes should a patient present in their clinic. Because the vast majority of dental procedures are performed outside an institutional environment, HAIs are less often reported, but there is, as discussed in Chapter 1, a risk of infection in every clinical setting. Much information aimed primarily at health professionals has sought to reduce the incidence of HAI and has emphasised the importance of procedures such as hand washing and barrier to personal protection discussed in Chapters 5 and 6. (Further information on HAI can be found at http://www.dh.gov.uk/en/Publichealth/Healthprotection/Healthcareacquiredinfection/index.htm.)

INFECTIOUS DISEASE BY ROUTE OF TRANSMISSION IN THE DENTAL SURGERY

There are three main routes by which infection can be transmitted in a dental practice:

1. Transmission by direct or indirect contact

2. Parenteral transmission via the bloodstream

3. Transmission via airborne and respiratory secretions

It is important to know the route of transmission of an infective agent as the infection control measures as set out in *standard precautions* are targeted at blocking the potential route of transmission (Figure 2.1). Problems often arise when the routes of transmission of new emerging infections pose a challenge to our standard precautions. For example, vCJD is difficult to denature and remove from instruments; hence, the contact route of transmission may not be blocked by our routine standard precautions and they have to be modified in the light of experimental evidence to reduce the risk of transmission.

Infection control in dentistry can be defined as a series of measures to block the route of transmission of pathogens within the dental surgery.

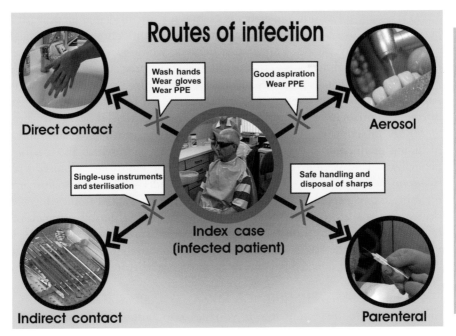

Figure 2.1 Routes of transmission of infection in the dental surgery and how they are blocked by standard infection control precautions (courtesy of Paul Morris).

Direct and indirect contact spread of infection

This is the most obvious and commonly appreciated mode of spread of infection by dental professionals. Contact spread is a direct spread from person to person, or indirectly via equipment, via contaminated fluids, or from food or objects such as towels.

Pathogens which have a risk of transmission by contact include the herpes group of viruses – herpes simplex virus (HSV), varicella zoster virus (VZV) and Epstein-Barr virus (EBV) a, hepatitis B virus (HBV) and the respiratory viruses. While we associate the spread of respiratory viruses with the spread by aerosol, it must not be forgotten that the patterns of transmission observed during nosocomial outbreaks of influenza suggest that large droplets from a patient with infection and contact (direct and indirect) are the most important and most likely routes of spread. Also, respiratory syncytial virus (RSV), a highly infectious respiratory virus, which causes outbreaks in hospitalised children is largely spread by direct contact. Many bacterial infections could potentially be transmitted by contact in the dental clinic but the one which causes most concern especially in oral surgery is *S. aureus*, in particular MRSA.

HSV is very infectious and patients commonly attend dental clinic with a herpes labialis or cold sore which can infect the dentist's fingers, resulting in an intensely painful lesion known as a herpetic whitlow. VZV which causes chicken pox and shingles is a risk to the fetus and pregnant women, and in many countries including the UK, dentists must be vaccinated if they have no natural immunity to prevent primary infection. This is to reduce the risk of infection to pregnant women from the health care worker (HCW).

MRSA infection is of concern because they are resistant to antibiotics including methicillin and other more common antibiotics such as oxacillin, penicillin and amoxicillin. About 25–30% of the population are colonised with *S. aureus* but only approximately 1% carry MRSA. MRSA occurs most frequently among persons in hospitals and health care facilities, and thus the dentist may be at greatest risks of becoming colonised during locum visits to patients in such institutions. The main mode of transmission of MRSA is via the hands of the HCW which may become contaminated by contact with either colonised or infected patients or from sites on their own body which are colonised or infected.

Community-acquired MRSA (CA-MRSA) is a different strain of MRSA that is easier to treat, and infects younger populations in the community and can, if left untreated, cause very serious disease. CA-MRSA primarily causes infection in athletes, children in day care and intravenous drug users, where there is close skin-to-skin contact and spread is encouraged by poor hygiene. (Further information on MRSA can be found at http://www.dh.gov.uk/en/AdvanceSearchResult/index.htm?searchTerms=MRSA.)

Prevention of person-to-person spread of infection

The primary source of spread from person to person is by hands and clothing and this route of infection is easily interrupted by hand washing and wearing of gloves (Figure 2.1), as outlined in Chapter 5.

Prevention of spread of infection from equipment

Equipment including dental instruments must be decontaminated between patients (Figure 2.1) or be discarded safely if they are designated single use, as outlined in Chapter 7. Impression materials should be disinfected to reduce the risk of infection of dental technicians and comply with regulation concerning the transport of infected material by postal services. Dental chairs and units must also be cleaned and disinfected between patients and this is facilitated by dividing the surgery into 'zones' of different levels of contamination, as outlined in Chapter 8.

Prevention of spread of infection by fluids

The dental unit waterlines are a potential source of the spread of infection by both aerosol and contact (Figure 2.1), and the management and method of reducing this risk is discussed in Chapter 9. Disinfectant and detergents must be stored in concentrated form according to the manufacturer's recommendation as they can become a source of infection by bacteria such as *Pseudomonas aeruginosa* which are resistant to some disinfectants and pose a risk to immunocompromised patients.

The transmission of infection via food is a major source of concern in society but should not be a risk in dentistry since no food should be taken in surgery and adequate kitchen facilities should be provided for staff.

Parenteral transmission of infection via the bloodstream

Many organisms are potentially transmissible in the occupational setting via percutaneous (sharps) (Figure 2.1) or mucocutaneous (mucous membrane/ broken skin) routes. The so-called *blood-borne viruses* (BBVs) are of primary concern. The BBVs which present most cross-infection hazard to HCWs are those associated with a carrier state with persistent replication of the virus in the human host and persistent viraemia. These include HIV and hepatitis B and C.

Hepatitis B virus

Hepatitis B is a blood-borne and sexually transmitted virus, a member of the Hepadnaviridae DNA family, which causes inflammation of the liver. Transmission usually occurs by unprotected sexual intercourse, intravenous drug misusers, sharing contaminated needles and from mother to baby at birth. Up to 90% of babies infected perinatally and around 5–10% of those infected as adults develop chronic carrier status. Many infected people have no symptoms, but others have a flu-like illness with nausea and jaundice. The persistence of the 'e'-antigen correlates with a high level of viral replication and increased infectivity. Hepatitis B becomes a chronic infection when the infection persists longer than 6 months and more than 350 million people worldwide have chronic infections. Hepatitis B is a significant problem for public health within the European region with over 1 million newly infected, 14 million chronically infected and 36 000 deaths annually attributed to HBV. The increase in prevalence is influenced by migration rates from high-incidence areas. Hepatitis B vaccine can prevent hepatitis B infection and the WHO has recommended, since 1991, universal hepatitis B vaccination of all newborns, children and/or adolescents against hepatitis B as well as vaccination of risk groups and the incidence of the disease has decreased significantly in countries that have implemented this policy. Vaccination has played a key role in prevention of HBV infection within the dental profession and is part of standard infection control policy, it is however not a substitute for the safe practices outlined in Chapter 3 and HCV with the other BBVs remains a risk of infection which cannot be mitigated by vaccination. (Useful website on HBV: http://www.hepatitisinfo.org/pdf/European_Policy_Recommendations.pdf.)

Hepatitis C virus

Hepatitis C is a blood-borne virus, a member of the Flaviviridae RNA virus family, which causes inflammation of the liver. Many people who are infected have no symptoms and are unaware that they are carrying the virus. There is a prevalence rate of about 3% (170 million) HCV infection worldwide, which varies widely between the countries, with 0.05% prevalence in UK blood donors, 1.03% (8.9 million) in Europe, 4.6% (21.3 million) in the Eastern Mediterranean and 5.3% (31.9 million) in Africa.

Chronic infection is defined as infection lasting longer than 6 months and up to 80% of infected people go on to develop chronic infection. People with chronic hepatitis C infection are at long-term risk of developing cirrhosis and liver cancer. The probability of transmission to an HCW following a needle-stick injury is estimated to be about 1.8%. A Scottish study (Roy *et al.*, 2003) of 880 dental staff found a prevalence of anti-HCV antibody of 0.1%, which is similar to that of the background population. Thus, the standard precautions applied by dentists are able to reduce the risk of HCV infection to acceptable levels, this despite the fact that there is no vaccine or prophylactic treatment available to prevent hepatitis C infection. (Useful website on HCV: http://www.who.int/mediacentre/factsheets/fs164/en/.)

Human immunodeficiency virus

The HIV is a retrovirus that infects cells of the human immune system, destroying or impairing their function. As the infection progresses, the immune system becomes weaker and at the most advanced stage of HIV infection develops acquired immunodeficiency syndrome (AIDS). The treatment of these infected patients requires the application of stringent standard infection controls to prevent cross-infection not only with the HIV virus but since these patients become more susceptible to opportunist infections they must be protected from infection from, for example, contaminated waterlines (see Chapter 9).

Most HIV transmission is by unprotected penetrative sexual intercourse, via infected blood mainly from injecting drug misuse and from mother to child. In the dental clinic, prevention focuses on safe handling of sharp instruments as outlined in Chapter 4 and training of staff. Even though the risk of infection with HIV is 100 times less than HBV for a similar exposure, the fear of the consequences of infection has often shaken dentists' confidence in their infection control measures to the extent that patients have in the past experienced difficulty obtaining dental treatment. It is important to be confident that standard infection control measures can reduce the risk of transmission of HIV to negligible levels. There are no recent reports of HIV acquired from dental practice either by the dentist or by the patient and only one report of a patient acquiring HIV from a dental procedure. (Useful website on HIV: http://www.dh.gov.uk/en/Publichealth/Healthimprovement/Sexualhealth/HIV/index.htm.)

Preventing BBV infection in the occupational setting

There were at least ten reported instances of transmission of HBV from dentist to patients before 1985 when the emergence of HIV led to improvements in infection control measures and since then there have been no recent cases of HBV transmission.

Even though the risk of transmission of BBV is significantly greater from patient to HCW than from HCW to patient, restrictions have been put on HCWs performing exposure-prone procedures (EPPs) to further reduce the risk of transmission of BBV from dentist to patient. EPPs are invasive procedures where there is a risk that injury to the HCW may result in exposure of the patient's open tissue to the blood of the worker. The vast majority of dental procedures are considered exposure prone, and unlike doctors those dentists who are unable to undertake EPP are effectively excluded from their profession (see Chapter 3).

An estimated 200 HCWs in the UK undertaking EPP are chronic carriers of HCV and to reduce the potential risk to patients, the Department of Health in England issued advice relating to the health clearance required for new HCWs in 2007. This guidance recommends that all new HCWs should have a standard health clearance check completed on appointment, which includes checks for TB disease/immunity, and are offered hepatitis B immunisation, with post-immunisation testing of response and the offer of tests for hepatitis C and HIV. Additional heath clearance is required for new HCWs who will perform EPPs. It means that the HCW must be non-infectious for HIV (antibody negative), hepatitis B (surface antigen negative or, if positive, e-antigen negative with a viral load of 10^3 genome equivalents/mL or less) and hepatitis C (antibody negative or, if positive, negative for hepatitis C RNA). These checks should be completed before confirmation of an appointment to an EPP's post, as the HCW will be ineligible if found to be infectious. This guidance is intended to reduce the risk of HCW-to-patient transmission of BBVs and TB and also to reduce patient notification exercises following incidents which tend to decrease public confidence in health care and require valuable resources.

Freedom from infection with BBVs is not an absolute requirement for those wishing to train as doctors since many career paths are available to doctors which do not require the performance of EPPs. However, this is not the case for all dentists, dental hygienists and therapists because EPPs are performed during training and practice; they require the additional health clearance and must be free from BBV infection.

Standard precautions should be adhered to in the clinical setting as outlined in Chapters 3 and 4. All HCWs should be immunised against hepatitis B infection and should be shown to have made a serological response to the vaccine. (Further information on immunisation can be found at http:// www.dh.gov.uk/en/Policyandguidance/Healthandsocialcaretopics/Greenbook/ DH_4097254. A useful website giving further information on all BBV is http:// www.hpa.org.uk/web/home.)

Spread of infection by airborne and respiratory secretions

Dental personnel are exposed to the risk of transmission of infection from the aerosols and fluid droplets generated by rotary instruments and ultrasonic scalers. The source of potential infection is the patient's saliva and blood and dental waterlines. The risk of occupational infection from waterlines is mainly from legionella and the management of waterlines is considered in Chapter 9.

Organisms which may be transmitted in aerosols include *Mycobacterium tuberculosis*, the respiratory viruses of the common cold, adenovirus and flu. Some of the herpes viruses such as chicken pox (VZV) and EBV can also be transmitted from secretions.

Tuberculosis

Tuberculosis (TB) is an increasing problem worldwide with over 1.7 billion infected and 60 million with active TB, which results in 3 million deaths annually. Since over 95% of the cases are in developing countries, many dentists do not perceive TB to be a risk in their practice. There are about 8000 cases per year in the UK, and this is on the increase. The reasons for the increase in prevalence of TB are due to social factors such as urban homelessness, in-travenous drug abuse and neglect of control programmes, and migration of populations from areas of high incidence. An important risk factor in dentistry is that patients with immune suppression due to AIDS can have TB reactivated and be a source of infection. Multi-drug-resistant TB is a great cause of concern and accounts for 2–3% of global cases of TB, but there are hot spots within Europe such as Estonia with 14% prevalence. Thus, the risk of transmission of TB is not confined only to the developing world and is a very serious public health concern.

There have been well-documented cases of transmission from patients to HCWs with reports of 56% of nurses in an AIDS ward being tuberculin positive. Increases in infections amongst HCWs of up to 50% were reported in New York over a 10-year period. Transmission of infection from dentist to patient is extremely rare, but there was a report of pulmonary TB developed in 15 patients following dental extractions by a community dentist with active TB in 1982. This potential risk of infection is the reason the UK recommends that all new HCWs should be assessed regarding personal or family history of TB and documentary evidence of tuberculin skin testing (or interferon-gamma testing) within the past 5 years and/or BCG scar check by an occupational health professional.

The prevention of aerosol and splatter transmission involves the application of standard precautions with emphasis on having a well-ventilated surgery (up to 8–10 air changes per hour), the control of aerosols by high-volume, externally ventilated aspiration, and wearing of masks, glasses and visors for personal protection, as discussed in Chapters 6 and 8. (A useful website on TB is www.nice.org.uk/CG033.)

Influenza

Influenza virus causes a respiratory illness with the symptoms of headache, fever, cough, sore throat, aching muscles and joints. The incubation period of human influenza ranges from 1 to 4 days (typically 2–3). Infectivity is proportional to symptom severity and maximal just after the onset of symptoms, and the period of communicability is typically up to 5 days after symptom onset in adults and 7 days in children, but can be considerably prolonged in immunocompromised patients. There are two main types of influenza virus with influenza type A usually causing more severe symptoms than influenza type B.

Because flu usually occurs every winter in the UK, it is referred to as *seasonal flu* and must be differentiated from *pandemic flu* and *avian flu*, which can occur at any time of year and which are discussed later under emerging pathogens. Health protection authorities in European countries monitor and record the incidence of seasonal flu and the uptake of seasonal flu vaccine. This information is used to guide the development of policies for protecting the population from influenza. They alert health professionals including dentists if there is increased incidence and encourage HCWs to get vaccinated.

Person-to-person spread of human influenza viruses is well established and, as mentioned previously, nosocomial outbreaks of influenza implicate direct spread by contact following contamination by large droplets. Airborne or fine-droplet spread can occur during the performance of aerosol-generating procedures, which is common in dentistry. Influenza viruses can survive on environmental surfaces, especially so on hard non-porous materials for up to 48 hours, and are easily deactivated by washing with soap and water or alcohol-based hand sanitisers and cleaning with normal household detergents.

Prevention of flu involves application of standard precautions with emphasis on hand hygiene, the wearing of personal protective equipment (PPE) as discussed in Chapter 5 and vaccination against the current strain of flu. (Useful website on flu: http://www.hpa.org.uk/infections/topics_az/influenza/pandemic/guidelines .htm.)

EMERGING AND RE-EMERGING PATHOGENS

Infections tend to become more prevalent when conditions allow for their transmission and may recede into the background over time as the conditions change. Table 2.1 presents a list of emerging infectious diseases listed by the National Institute of Health in the USA. Fortunately, not many of these impact on dentistry. Infections such as caused by *Escherichia coli*, *Salmonella* and *Clostridium botulinum* are of concern in the food industry, while multi-drug-resistant organisms apart from MRSA, as discussed above, cause a risk of transmission primarily in hospitals where there are susceptible patients and frequent antibiotic use.

Emerging pathogens are of importance in the dental clinic for two reasons. Firstly, they challenge our infection control and prevention protocols and ask the question, 'Is there a risk of transmission of this infection in the dental surgery?' Secondly, 'new infections' can shake the confidence of the public and the dental team and therefore we need to educate the dental profession regarding

Table 2.1 Emerging infectious disease

Anthrax
Antimicrobial resistance[a]
Botulism
Campylobacteriosis
Dengue fever
Ehrlichiosis
E. coli 0157 infection
Flu (influenza)[a]
Group A Streptococcal infections[a]
Hepatitis[a]
Lyme disease
Plague
Prion diseases[a]
SARS
Salmonellosis/*Salmonella*
Shigellosis/*Shigella*
Smallpox
Tuberculosis[a]
Tularemia
West Nile virus[a]

[a] Diseases that are a possible risk of transmission in dentistry.

COMMUNICABLE DISEASES IN THE DENTAL SURGERY

the disease so that they can perform the risk assessment, discussed previously, and reassure the dental team and the public that dental treatment is safe.

Why do infections emerge?

Changes in climate, agricultural practices, urbanisation, antibiotic selection and health status of the population (immunosuppression or famine) can assist in the emergence of an infection. Increased access to travel and migration of people has a strong association with the spread of infection. The Black Death was associated with increased travel by ships and new risks are posed by increased travel by air. There were 104.8 million international arrivals in the UK in 2006 with 12.9 million being from outside the EU. This is the reason why information on recent travel outside the country is important when detecting emerging infections as the patient may have contacted the infection abroad and shown symptoms only upon returning home.

The impact of emerging infections on dentistry

Emerging infections in the past, which have impacted on dental treatment, were HBV, HCV and HIV. These BBV changed the face of modern dentistry and led to many of the improvements in infection control which we discuss in this book. They can no longer be considered emerging, but the reaction of the profession to each as it emerged may be a lesson for the future and explain our present approach to more recent emerging infections. When HBV and later HIV emerged, the profession adopted what is known as the *identify–refer paradigm*; i.e. we sought to identify patients with the infection and treat them with enhanced infection control measures above that of patients who did not 'apparently' pose a risk of these infections. The difficulty with this approach is that, as discussed previously, we cannot identify carriers of HCV and HBV, for example. As scientific evidence advanced our knowledge of these viruses, we incorporated necessary precautions into universal or standard precautions and moved to the *universal-risk paradigm*. The profession treated patients with these infections in the same way as other patients confident that the diseases posed no risk of infection to dental staff or other patients.

How have the emerging infections such as vCJD, pandemic flu and SARS (severe acute respiratory syndrome) impacted on the practice of dentistry?

Pandemic influenza and avian flu

Pandemics arise when a new virus emerges which is capable of spreading in the worldwide population. This was the situation during the influenza pandemic of 1918–1919, when a completely new influenza virus subtype (influenza A/H1N1) emerged and spread around the globe in waves over a 2-year period, killing an estimated 40–50 million people. There have been two subsequent influenza pandemics, in 1957 and 1968. There are concerns that the currently circulating avian influenza A/H5N1 strain may give rise to the next pandemic influenza virus.

The precautions required in the event of an outbreak of pandemic or avian flu are similar to those for seasonal flu described above. The only difference is that there is a national contingency plan for the outbreak and HCW will be instructed when to present for vaccination and acquisition of antiviral drugs if required. Strict adherence to standard infection control practice, in particular PPE and hand washing, is essential. One of the anti-flu drugs that are available is oseltamivir (Tamiflu), which is an orally administered neuraminidase inhibitor. It is licenced for the treatment of influenza A and B within 48 hours of the onset of symptoms in those aged above 1 year and post-exposure prevention in those aged 13 years and over when influenza is circulating in the community. Tamiflu is pre-packed in adult treatment courses – 75 mg twice daily for 5 days. The recommended dose for children between 24 and 40 kg body weight is 60 mg twice daily.

Severe acute respiratory syndrome

SARS is caused by a coronavirus (CoV) of the same family as the common cold virus. It emerged in China in 2003 and resulted in 8437 probable cases with 813 deaths. The death rate ranged from 1 to 50% of cases, being greater in those over 65 years. What alarmed the world community was its rate of spread and it was termed a *super-spreader* as it spread rapidly around the world from China to Canada. SARS virus is not as infectious as influenza and requires close contact but has a higher mortality. It has multiple sites of replication in the body and is spread by respiratory secretions and by faeces. The infectivity increases as the disease progresses and reaches a maximum around day 10 when the patient is very seriously ill. This is the reason why about one-third of cases were HCWs. Dentists were at less risk than other HCWs as patients would be unlikely to present for treatment during these peak infectious periods unless the dentist was called to an acute ward in a hospital.

There are contingency plans in place should another outbreak occur, and dentist will be informed should the need arise. Key issues arising in relation to infection control are a good medical history of travel, etc., PPE, hand washing and being vaccinated against the flu, so that if HCWs displayed flu-like symptoms during an SARS outbreak the suspicion would be that it was SARS and not seasonal flu.

Variant Creutzfeldt–Jakob disease and transmissible spongiform encephalopathy agents

Human cases of vCJD linked to consuming foods tainted with BSE (bovine spongiform encephalopathy) were first diagnosed in 1995 with the epidemic peaking in 2000 with 6 deaths per quarter in mid-2000, declining to a current incidence of about 1.2 deaths per quarter. The total number of deaths from vCJD in Europe is approximately 250, the majority of whom (163 cases; figures up to March 2008) were in the UK. In contrast to SARS and pandemic flu it has killed very few people and has not spread rapidly around the globe, yet this disease has had a major impact on how we practice dentistry in the UK.

vCJD is not caused by a living entity but is spread by a 'rogue protein' molecule called *prion* and belongs to a group of diseases known as TSE (transmissible spongiform encephalopathy). While CJD prions are confined to the central nervous system (CNS), vCJD prions are detected in the CNS and in the peripheral nervous system and lymphoid tissues. Four cases of transmission of vCJD via blood transfusion were reported in 2003–2004 in the UK. Each of the cases had received blood from donors who appeared well at the time of donation, but later died of vCJD. Prions have also been identified in the trigeminal ganglion and tonsils from patients at postmortem. The incubation period for the disease from infection is of the order 4–40 years (mean 10–15 years).

Thus, we are confronted with the problem of how to quantify risk when a disease may not emerge for 15 years. We can make an initial risk assessment of the likelihood of prion's transmission occurring during dental treatment. As with all emerging pathogens our knowledge base is in its infancy and continues to evolve as our understanding grows. Abrasion of the lingual tonsil is considered a highly unlikely event during routine dental treatment but could occur during maxillofacial procedures. Dental pulp, which is composed of vascular and peripheral nerve tissue, was shown to be infected with vCJD in animal studies. Similarly, the dental pulp of individuals sub-clinically infected with vCJD may be infectious, although the level of infectivity is unknown.

Secondly, how can we kill an entity which is not alive? This has led the profession to return again to the identify–refer paradigm, since there are thought to be very few cases of patients at risk of transmitting this infection. Initial figures published in 2004 based on testing 12 000 tonsils for vCJD found three positive cases. Extrapolation of the figures indicated that approximately 3800 people are incubating the disease in the UK, but the latest projected figures suggest that the figure may be closer to 6000 carriers. Many of these people may remain as long-term asymptomatic infectious carriers of the disease, posing a potential risk for cross-infection to others when they use health care services.

The possible routes of transmission are by surgical instruments and by blood products. This has focused dentists and health professionals on how to prevent transmission by contact with dental instruments. The challenge to standard infection control precautions posed by vCJD was, 'Can the existing instrument decontamination protocols reduce the risk of transmission of the prion sufficiently?' There was evidence that the routine autoclave holding time of 3 minutes at 134°C would not guarantee inactivation of the prion infective agent. Therefore, the emphasis shifted to adequate pre-sterilization washing of instruments and quality control of the decontamination process as outlined in Chapter 7.

The Department of Health in England stated in 2003 that 'the risk of transmission from dental instruments is very low provided optimal standards of infection control and decontamination are maintained'. This has been the source of much debate as the definition of 'optimal decontamination standards' can vary greatly between countries. Much of the changes and standards outlined in this book in relation to instrument decontamination and increased use of single-use instruments, outlined in Chapter 7, have been with the aim of improving these processes to a level that instruments used on patients with vCJD can be safely reused on other patients and thus these patients can be included in the universal-risk paradigm and treated in the same way that other patients are under standard infection control protocols.

West Nile virus

West Nile virus first appeared in New York City in the summer of 1999 and by the end of the summer 62 patients were hospitalised and 7 were dead. The infection subsequently spread to Canada and over 250 patients had died in the USA. The infection is spread by a mosquito, but can be spread by transfusion and potentially medical instruments. Thus, it poses no great threat to dentists or their patients beyond that of the community, but since we know the potential route of transmission via blood we can successfully block these by the application of standard infection control practice.

The bottom line is that no matter what new or emerging infections arise in the future so long as we have information of their routes of transmission and are assured that our standard infection control policies and protocols are able to block these routes, our patients and our staff are safe. If there is uncertainty in this regard the profession will take on board scientific evidence, perform a risk assessment and adjust our protocols to cope with the new situation. We therefore live in a dynamic changing world and the topics outlined in this book should make you better able to meet this challenging future.

REFERENCES AND WEBSITES

Roy, K., Kennedy, C., Bagg, J., Cameron, S., Hunter, I. and Taylor, M. (2003). Hepatitis C infection among dental personnel in the West of Scotland, UK. *Journal of Hospital Infection*, 55, 73–76.

Further reading

MRSA: Available at http://www.dh.gov.uk/en/AdvanceSearchResult/index.htm?search Terms=MRSA.

CA-MRSA: Available at http://www.cdc.gov/ncidod/dhqp/ar_mrsa_ca.html.

HBV: Available at http://www.hepatitisinfo.org/pdf/European_Policy_Recommendations. pdf.

Vaccination: Available at http://www.dh.gov.uk/en/Policyandguidance/Healthandsocialc aretopics/Greenbook/DH_4097254.

HCV: Available at http://www.who.int/mediacentre/factsheets/fs164/en/.

HIV: Available at http://www.dh.gov.uk/en/Publichealth/Healthimprovement/Sexualheal th/HIV/index.htm.

BBV: Available at http://www.hpa.org.uk/web/home.

TB: Clinical diagnosis and management of tuberculosis, and measures for its prevention and control – National Institute for Health and Clinical Excellence (NICE) tuberculosis clinical guideline. Available at www.nice.org.uk/CG033.

Department of Health/Health Protection Division/General Health Protection (2007). *Health Clearance for Tuberculosis, Hepatitis B, Hepatitis C and HIV: New Health-care Workers*. Department of Health – Publications and statistics.htm.

Influenza: Available at http://www.hpa.org.uk/infections/topics_az/influenza/pandemic/ guidelines.htm.

Emerging Infections: Available at http://www3.niaid.nih.gov/healthscience/healthtopics/ emerging/default.htm.

vCJD: Available at http://www.hpa.org.uk/webw/HPAweb&Page&HPAwebAutoList Name/Page/1191942152861.

COMMUNICABLE DISEASES IN THE DENTAL SURGERY

Chapter 3

Occupational health and immunisation

PROVISION OF OCCUPATIONAL HEALTH

In this chapter, we will examine building a culture of safety, pre-employment health assessments, immunisation, exposure-prone procedures (EPPs) and health clearance, all of which contribute to staying healthy in the dental practice. In the working environment, members of the dental team are exposed to a number of hazardous substances such as natural rubber latex and disinfectants as well as microbial pathogens.

So, if you want to stay healthy in the dental practice then the first stage is to identify where the major occupational health hazards might lie.

Risk activities in dentistry that relate to occupational health include:

- Sharps injuries and exposure to blood-borne virus (see Chapter 4)

- Respiratory infections from inhaling contaminated aerosols from dental unit waterlines, e.g. Legionnaires' disease and Pontiac fever, exacerbation of asthma by endotoxins and Gram-negative bacteria (see Chapters 6 and 9)

- Exposure to respiratory aerosols and secretions from infected patients, e.g. tuberculosis (TB), influenza, varicella, measles, rubella (see Chapter 6)

- Eye and skin infections, e.g. herpetic whitlow, impetigo, conjunctivitis (see Chapter 5)

- Hypersensitive reactions affecting skin and respiratory system, e.g. natural rubber latex, methyl methacrylate, glutaraldehyde (see Chapter 6)

- Mercury toxicity (see Chapter 10)

- Exposure to irradiation (outside the remit of this book)

Health and safety law requires the dentist to implement necessary measures to protect all members of the dental team and patients from such risks as far as is reasonably practicable.

BUILDING A CULTURE OF SAFETY

One of the main strategies for combating transmission of infection from person to person within the practice is to develop a culture of safety. Safe working practices, compliance with infection control policies, reporting injuries and near misses and effective management form the backbone of a dental practice safety culture. Personal protective equipment (PPE; see Chapter 6), sharps safety devices, immunisation and post-exposure prophylaxis (see Chapter 5) provide the protective defences against transmission of infection. Figure 3.1 illustrates how all these factors could come together to create a culture of safety within the dental practice.

This approach requires a commitment from the whole dental team if it is to be successful. Everyone in the dental team including students and trainees has an important contribution to make. Some of the steps the dental practice can take to create a safety culture are shown in Table 3.1.

Accidents such as sharps injuries will occur in the practice, however well it is run, but it is important to try and understand why an accident or a near miss occurred to prevent it from happening again. Mistakes and accidents tend not to be random mishaps but to fall into recurrent patterns, referred to as *error traps*. The same set of circumstances can provoke similar errors or accidents regardless of the member of staff or student who is involved. To be effective, cross-infection prevention necessitates looking beyond the simple explanation that it was someone's fault and attempt to answer the much harder question as

OCCUPATIONAL HEALTH AND IMMUNISATION

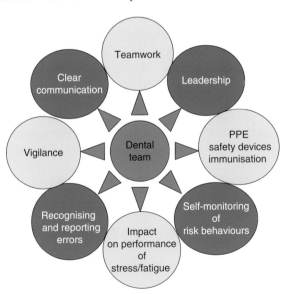

Figure 3.1 How the dental team can work together to build a safety culture.

Table 3.1 Steps involved in creating a practice safety culture

A safety culture is created through:
• Actions the practice management takes to improve patient and dental health care personnel safety
• All the members of the dental team participating in safety planning and infection control protocol development
• Influence of group norms regarding acceptable safety practices
• Routine and occupational immunisation, post-exposure prophylaxis, availability of appropriate protective equipment and training in its correct use
• Induction training and socialisation process for new dental personnel or students

to 'why' the error occurred in the first place. There is seldom a single reason. Breakdowns in the practices infection control management and defences can arise from two main causes:

• Active failures

• Latent conditions

Active failures are unsafe acts committed by frontline people in direct contact with the patient. Their impact is usually instantaneous and breaches the integrity of the practice 'defences'. In many cases, such acts have a causal history that extends back in time. The case scenario examples given below show how active and latent failures can combine and stack up with serious long-term consequences:

Example of an active failure: During a surgical extraction on a patient with hepatitis B the suture needle is covered by a bloody swab and both are discarded into a waste sack. The needle punctures the plastic and the cleaner receives a sharps injury when she empties the pedal bin.

Example of a series of latent failures: The cleaner had not been vaccinated against hepatitis B. She was a temporary cleaner from an agency and was covering for the practices regular cleaner who was on holiday. Nobody at the agency or the dental practice had checked if she was vaccinated against hepatitis B. Three months later she was diagnosed with hepatitis B. She worked at night after the practice had closed and had not reported the accident. As there was no record of the incident in the accident book, she was unable to prove where she acquired the infection from and was unable to make an insurance claim to which she would have been entitled.

Table 3.2 Where latent failures could occur in dental practice

Poor design of surgery and equipment
Ineffective training
Inadequate supervision
Ineffective communications
Uncertainties in roles and responsibilities

Whereas latent failures arise from decisions made on the design, procedures and management within the practice (see Table 3.2) or may relate to decisions taken outside the dental practice by third parties, such as equipment and instrument manufacturers, or government health authorities. Latent or delayed failures can remain dormant for many years until they combine with active failures and other local triggers to create an opportunity for an accident. If the dental practice's infection-control policy and 'defences' function as intended, the results of the unsafe act are caught and the effects limited. If not, the accident could have tragic and long-term consequences (see the examples above). To prevent latent failures causing repeated incidents they require proactive rather than reactive responses on behalf of the dental team.

A way of highlighting active and latent failures in the dental practice is to use root cause analysis. Staff and students working on the 'frontline' are usually in the best position to identify issues and solution. The aim of a root cause analysis is to determine:

- What happened?

- Why did it happen?

- What can you do to prevent it from happening again?

ORGANISING STAFF HEALTH IN YOUR PRACTICE

Pre-employment health assessment

All new employees in the dental practice (including trainees, students, part-time and agency staff) should undergo a pre-employment health assessment which includes checking their vaccination history, flagging up any additional pre-employment vaccines they require based on a risk assessment of the duties they will be performing in the post, e.g. does the person have direct or close clinical contact with the patient. Do they perform EPPs?

Everyone working in the practice has a duty of care towards the patients, which includes taking reasonable precautions to protect them from

OCCUPATIONAL HEALTH AND IMMUNISATION

communicable diseases. This can be achieved by appropriate immunisation against vaccine-preventable diseases. But immunisation should never be regarded as a substitute for safe working. Immunisation directly protects the individual and indirectly protects their family and friends, colleagues and vulnerable patients. Preventing communicable infections, e.g. influenza, promotes efficient running of the dental practice and reduces disruptions caused by the staff absent on sick leave.

Immunisation programme and staff health records

The dentists as employers need to be able to demonstrate that they have an effective employee immunisation programme in place. It is normally recommended that the practice nominates a person to coordinate the administration of staff health and the reporting and recording of accidents and near misses within the practice. The practice should keep a confidential record of health clearance records including hepatitis B antibody test results and occupational immunisation schedules. Include an alerting system in the records as this helps ensure that the records are contemporary and that all members of the dental team are up to date with booster vaccinations, although it is strongly recommended that immunisation programmes are managed by the local occupational health services. The following information will need to be recorded:

- Sharps injuries, accidents and incidents and near misses
- Pre-employment health clearance
- Date for booster vaccination

We know that underreporting of a sharps and a splash injury is common. It is helpful if the health coordinator in the dental practice understands the reasons why injuries are not reported or recorded and addresses barriers to reporting that apply in their own practice.

Failure to report accidents or near misses is due to:

- Fear of being accused of negligence
- Fear of being labelled accident prone
- Reputation with peers
- Conflict of loyalty to patient or practice (bear silent witness)
- Fear of subsequent medical treatment (sharps injuries)
- Lack of understanding of purpose of accident reporting

A wise man said, 'To err is human'. High-risk industries with the potential for disastrous accidents such as nuclear power and airlines are pioneers in the field of industrial safety. Their excellent safety record is based on a non-blame approach, with the emphasis firmly on prevention, not punishment. Both industries have found this to be the best method to encourage reporting of incidents and near misses by their staff.

IMMUNISATION REQUIREMENTS FOR DENTISTRY

In the UK, it is recommended that all health care staff are up to date with routine vaccinations against tetanus, diphtheria, polio, and measles, mumps and rubella (MMR; Salisbury *et al.*, *Immunisation Against Infectious Disease – 'The Green Book'*, 2006). Clinical staff and students who have direct contact with patient or body fluids will require additional vaccinations for hepatitis B, TB (BCG vaccine) and varicella (if non-immune) (see Table 3.3). Annual vaccination in the autumn against seasonal influenza is strongly recommended for all members of the dental team. Increasing attention is being directed towards improving influenza vaccination uptake rates in all health care personnel. Antiviral drugs are available for the treatment of seasonal influenza, but in the UK, NHS doctors are permitted to prescribe the drugs only when the number of cases per week exceeds a Department of Health specified threshold. Avian flu and pandemic influenza are discussed in Chapter 2.

PROTECTING WOMEN OF CHILDBEARING AGE

Varicella

Women of childbearing age working in the dental practice should protect themselves from infections that can cause damage to the fetus during pregnancy, e.g. rubella, varicella and syphilis. Antenatal anonymous screening results collected in 2007 showed that 2.5% of pregnant women were non-immune to rubella. A vaccine capable of protecting against rubella has been available since the 1970s in Europe, but has not been universally available in resource-poor countries. Poor vaccine coverage in the UK is in part due to unsubstantiated fears of an increased risk of autism in infants receiving the MMR. In recent years, there have been outbreaks of mumps and measles amongst young adults including dental students who were too old to receive the MMR vaccine, but did not have an opportunity to develop natural immunity. The World Health Organization (WHO) recommends two doses of a measles-containing vaccine (see www.who.int/mediacentre/factsheets/fs286/en/). See Table 3.3 for recommendations on vaccination with MMR and serological testing.

OCCUPATIONAL HEALTH AND IMMUNISATION

Table 3.3 Recommended occupational immunisation

Disease	Occupational route of spread	Pre- or post-immunisation serological testing	Type of vaccine	Dosing schedule in health care workers	Occupational immunisation recommendation
Varicella (chickenpox, shingles)	Respiratory droplets or direct contact with blisters, contaminated clothing	Pretesting	Varicella live attenuated vaccine	2 doses 4–8 weeks apart	All non-immune clinical staff
Tuberculosis	Respiratory droplets	Pretesting; Mantoux test	BCG; live attenuated, derived from Mycobacterium bovis	Single dose	Clinical staff (unvaccinated, tuberculin-negative individuals aged under 35 years; over 35 years job-based risk assessment)
Hepatitis B	Sharps injuries and blood exposure of mucous membranes or non-intact skin	Post-immunisation	Inactivated	3 or 4 doses; reinforcing vaccination at 5 years or as prophylaxis following sharps/mucosal injury	No evidence of previous immunisation or disease; clinical staff
Mumps, measles, rubella	Droplet spread	N/A	MMR, live attenuated	Two doses	Clinical staff unless written evidence of two doses of MMR, or positive antibody tests for measles and rubella
Influenza	Aerosols, droplets and direct contact	N/A	Trivalent, containing two subtypes of influenza A and one type B virus	Single dose	Clinical and reception staff

Two live vaccines should not be given simultaneously, e.g. MMR, varicella and BCG, but should be given 4 weeks apart. Natural interferon is produced in response to a live vaccine. If a second live vaccine is given during this response period, the interferon may prevent replication of the second vaccine virus and the antibody response and vaccine effectiveness may be reduced.

Varicella immunisation

Chickenpox is caused by the varicella zoster virus and is highly infectious. The infection can occur at any age but is more common in children. However, disease in adults tends to be more severe. The primary infection presents initially with itchy blisters on the skin that later scab and may cause scarring. The virus eventually becomes latent in the sensory ganglion (nerve cells), but can reactivate later in life as shingles (herpes zoster) resulting in a painful, vesicular (blistering) skin rash. Vesicles whether in the primary or the reactivation secondary form of the disease contain virus and are infectious.

In pregnant women, chickenpox infection during the first 20 weeks of pregnancy can occasionally cause damage to the fetus; fortunately, this is an uncommon occurrence. The newborn baby may also be infected if the mother develops chickenpox during the perinatal period. Perinatal chickenpox in the newborn is associated with a high death rate if the mother is infected 5 days before the baby is born or 2 days after delivery. This is thought to be due to the newborn baby not receiving transplacental antibodies from the mother and the immaturity of the baby's immune system.

Recommendations for varicella vaccination

Approximately, 10% of the population have no immunity to chickenpox. Varicella immunisation is now recommended for non-immune members of the dental team who have direct patient contact. Vaccination protects both susceptible health care workers and vulnerable patients who might acquire chickenpox from an infected member of staff. Staff or students who have no previous history of chickenpox or shingles should have a blood test to check their immunity. If there is a definite history of chickenpox or shingles the person can be considered to be immune. Those who are seronegative (with no antibody evidence of immunity) are recommended to be vaccinated. They should receive two doses of the live attenuated vaccine 4–8 weeks apart. Routine post-serological testing is not advised. Varicella vaccine is contraindicated in pregnancy and as a precaution should be avoided for 3 months post-vaccination. Surveillance of inadvertent vaccination of pregnant women in the USA has not, however, identified any special risk to the fetus.

Rubella

Rubella is a mild disease caused by a togavirus; it is spread by droplet transmission. It may begin with a mild prodromal illness involving a low-grade fever, malaise and mild conjunctivitis. The erythematous (red) rubella rash on the ears, face and neck can easily be missed as it is transitory. Incubation period is 14–21 days, and the person is infectious from 1 week before symptoms appear to 4 days after the onset of the rash. Infection in pregnancy may result in foetal loss or in congenital rubella syndrome (cataracts and other eye defects, deafness, cardiac abnormalities, microcephaly, inflammatory lesions of brain, liver, lungs and bone marrow). Infection in the first 8–10 weeks of pregnancy results in damaging up to 90% of surviving infants, with multiple defects being common. The risk of damage in the later stages of pregnancy declines and except for deafness, foetal damage is rare after 16 weeks. In the UK and elsewhere, rubella immunisation was routinely used to immunise prepubertal girls and non-immune women of childbearing age to prevent rubella infection in pregnancy. Selective vaccination of teenage girls ceased in 1996. This has been replaced with the MMR vaccine, which is administered to infants and adults of both sexes with the long-term aim of eradicating these diseases from the population. MMR is given in over 100 countries, including those in the European Union. In Finland, a two-dose MMR schedule was introduced in 1982. As a result of persistently high vaccine coverage of the population, indigenous MMR was eliminated from Finland in 1994 and has not returned.

Syphilis

In the last few years, syphilis has seen a re-emergence due to outbreaks originating in major cities across Europe. The majority of cases are in men who have sex with men, though smaller numbers of heterosexual women including pregnant women have also been infected. Syphilis can cross the placenta and infect the fetus. Anonymous antenatal serological testing in the UK in 2007 showed that 0.13% of pregnant women were treponemal antibody-positive.

Oral sex was identified as the route of transmission in some of the notified cases. Dentists should refer any patients with suspicious lesions suggestive of either primary syphilis (presenting as a chancre – an indurated ulcer) or secondary syphilis (presenting as oral ulceration and/or mucosal lesions) to their local sexual health clinic. Syphilis is most infectious during the early stages of the disease; although the overwhelming majority of cases are spread by sexual contact, syphilis can be spread by touching an active lesion present on the lips or oral mucosa. Surgical gloves provide an effective barrier to transmission. *Treponema pallidum*, the causative agent of syphilis, is carried in the blood and an accidental direct inoculation via a needle-stick injury can result in syphilis of the fingers. Antibiotic prophylaxis is available following occupational exposure and prompt advice should be sought from the local Occupational Health Department or a general medical practitioner.

WHO SHOULD BE IMMUNISED AGAINST HEPATITIS B?

All dental health care personnel, students and others (such as domestic staff) who have contact with blood/body fluids, clinical waste and sharps in the course of their duties should have received and completed a hepatitis B immunisation course. Since the introduction of routine hepatitis B vaccine for clinical staff and students, the number of cases of occupationally acquired hepatitis B has fallen dramatically.

There are two classes of products available for occupational immunisation against hepatitis B: a vaccine that confers active immunity, and hepatitis B immunoglobulin (HBIG) that provides passive and temporary immunity for those at high risk of infection following a sharps injury. Post-exposure prophylaxis against hepatitis B is discussed in Chapter 4.

Hepatitis B vaccine

Hepatitis B vaccine is prepared from yeast cells using recombinant DNA technology. As the vaccine contains inactivated virus it is very safe and is incapable of causing hepatitis. A standard vaccine course consists of three immunisations that stimulate the production of specific antibodies to hepatitis B surface antigen (HBsAg). Approximately, 10–15% of adults fail to respond to three doses of vaccine or respond poorly. Poor responses are mostly associated with age over 40 years, obesity, alcohol intake, smoking and immunosuppression. Vaccine is ineffective in patients with acute hepatitis B, and is not necessary for individuals known to have markers of current (HBsAg) or evidence of past hepatitis B infection.

Antibody response to the vaccine is measured at 1–2 months after completing the course of immunisation to ensure that an adequate antibody (hepatitis B surface antibody titre (HBsAb) ≥ 100 IU/mL) response has been mounted and the titre recorded. Antibody responses vary widely between individuals. In the UK, anti-HBs levels above 100 mIU/mL are accepted as evidence of a good immune response, although titres of ≥ 10 mIU/mL are generally accepted as offering protect against infection.

Maximum antibody titres are usually found 1 month after completing the course with a rapid decline over the next 12 months and thereafter the titre falls more slowly. Immunological memory ensures that protection against infection is sustained even though the circulating concentration of antibodies declines with time. However, recent evidence suggests that not all individuals may respond in this way and the full duration of protection afforded by hepatitis B vaccine has yet to be completely established. Therefore, dental personnel at continuing risk of infection should be offered a single booster (reinforcing) dose of vaccine 5 years after the primary immunisation. A further assessment of antibody levels is not indicated. If a reinforcing dose is given before 5 years for post-exposure prophylaxis then a second reinforcing dose at 5 years is not required.

Poor responders and non-responders

Poor responders with an antibody response of between 10 and 100 IU/mL should be offered an additional dose of vaccine as this may improve the initial antibody titre. They should also receive the standard reinforcing dose at 5 years as recommended above.

Non-responders to hepatitis B vaccine

An antibody level below 10 IU/mL is classified as a non-response to vaccine, and testing for markers of current or past infection is a good clinical practice. Other vaccine non-responders may have natural immunity to hepatitis B due to past infection from which they have fully recovered and cleared the virus or alternatively they may be asymptomatic carriers of hepatitis B. Both groups do not respond to the vaccine and for employment health clearance it is essential to determine which category the dental health care worker or student falls into. True non-responders are normally offered a repeat course of immunisation. This is followed by retesting 1–4 months after the second course. If they fail to mount an adequate antibody response, and remain non-responders, they will require prompt referral to the local Accident and Emergency Department/Occupational Health Department following a needle-stick injury for assessment, and if required hepatitis B immunoglobulin.

BCG vaccine

TB is caused by infection with *Mycobacterium tuberculosis*. The most common form is pulmonary TB, which accounts for almost 60% of all cases in the UK, although it can affect almost every part of the body. General symptoms include fever, loss of appetite, weight loss, night sweats and a persistent productive cough, accompanied by bloodstained sputum. In the Europe, most cases are acquired through the respiratory route. TB is not an inevitable result of infection with the bacterium. There are three possible responses: The initial infection may be eliminated by the immune system; or remains latent in the body and reactivates if the individual becomes immunosuppressed at a later date; or causes active TB. Up until 2005, school children were vaccinated against TB at the age of 12–14 years. This programme has now ceased and been replaced with a targeted, risk-based immunisation protocol for susceptible neonates. Studies examining the effectiveness of BCG vaccine from across the world have reported wide variations from no protection to 70–80% protection in the UK schoolchildren. The vaccine is less effective in preventing the pulmonary form of the disease which is the predominant form in adults. Vaccine protection may wane over time, but is normally considered effective for about 10–15 years.

Health care workers are more likely than the general population to come into contact with someone with TB. BCG vaccination is recommended for dental health care personnel and students who have direct or close contact with patients. Unvaccinated, tuberculin-negative individuals aged under 35 years are recommended to receive BCG. Those entering the profession over the age of 35 years should seek specialist occupational advice and assessment as there is limited data on the protection afforded by BCG vaccine when it is given to adults aged 35 years or over.

OCCUPATIONAL HEALTH AND IMMUNISATION

HEALTH CLEARANCE AND THE CONSEQUENCES OF BLOOD-BORNE VIRUS INFECTION

All staff and students entering the health service for the first time or rejoining after a period of absence are obliged to complete statutory pre-employment health checks. Each person is individually assessed based on the clinical procures outlined in their job description or training programme. Those undertaking EPPs or having direct patient contact will require additional health screening tests. The purpose of these recommendations is to restrict health care workers infected with blood-borne virus (BBV) from working in the clinical areas where their infection may pose a risk to patients in their care.

Exposure-prone procedures –'bleed back'

Most routine dental treatments are classified as EPP.

An EPP is defined as a clinical procedure where there is a possibility of unrecognised bleed back into the patient's open tissues. The term is applied to all clinical procedures where hands or fingertips coming into contact with sharps

Table 3.4 Classification of exposure-prone procedures

Category	Associated risk	Example of dental procedure
1	**Lowest risk** of bleed back as the worker's hands are usually visible outside the mouth	Giving a local anaesthetic
2	**Intermediate risk** of bleed back, hands are partially visible but if bleed back occurs it would be recognised and acted on quickly	Extraction of a tooth
3	**Greatest risk** of significant injury and unrecognised bleed back	Osteotomy

may not be completely visible at all times. Sharps include needle tips, sharp instruments or sharp tissues such as teeth or bone spicules.

EPPs are classified into three broad categories based on the degree of visibility of the hands and the risk of significant sharps injury occurring during the procedure (see Table 3.4). Most routine dental treatment performed in primary care falls within categories 1 and 2, but certain maxillofacial surgery procedures are defined as category 3. Taking an extraoral radiograph, examination of the mouth with a mouth mirror, taking impressions and fitting full dentures in a totally edentulous patient are not considered to be exposure prone.

HEALTH CLEARANCE

Standard health checks

It is current policy in the NHS to screen all new entrants and those rejoining the health service including dental students on appointment for (Department of Health, 2007):

- TB immunity (evidence of tuberculin skin testing or interferon-gamma testing and/or BCG scar check by an occupational health professional)

- Offer of hepatitis B immunisation, with post-immunisation testing of response

- Offer of testing for hepatitis C and HIV, in the context of reminding health care workers of their professional responsibilities in relation to serious communicable diseases

Dental health care personnel and students for whom hepatitis B vaccination is contraindicated, who decline vaccination or who are non-responders to vaccine:

- Should be restricted from performing EPPs unless shown to be non-infectious (i.e. negative for hepatitis B surface antigen)
- Periodic retesting may need to be considered

Additional health checks

All health care workers who perform EPPs (such as dentists/therapists/hygienists/dental students) will also need to have 'additional health checks' that should be completed prior to confirmation of appointment or training place as the health care worker will be ineligible if found to be infectious. They should be free from infection with HIV and active TB. In addition, they must comply with the guidelines set out below for hepatitis B virus (HBV) and hepatitis C virus (HCV) bloodstream viral load. These viral titres reflect both threshold levels of virus needed to initiate infection and innovations in antiviral treatment.

Additional health clearance

The health care workers or students must be non-infectious for:

- HIV antibody-negative
- Hepatitis B surface antigen-negative (or, if positive, e-antigen negative with a viral load of 10^3 genome equivalents/mL or less)
- Hepatitis C antibody-negative (or if positive, negative for hepatitis C RNA)

Testing is a one-off and relies on the current obligation for health care workers to seek confidential professional advice, if they believe that they may subsequently have been exposed to a BBV or TB.

To some dental health care personnel, this guidance may appear draconian and differs from recommendations in the USA where HIV seropositive dental staff are permitted to provide the full range of dental treatment for their patients. HIV transmission during clinical procedures is 100 times less common than that of hepatitis B and 80 times less than hepatitis C. Since HIV was first diagnosed in the developing world, there has only been one proven case of HIV-positive dentist who infected their patients. The case in question is the much-publicised 1990 Acer case in Florida, USA. The dentist infected six of his patients. Even after extensive investigations costing $4 million, the method by which HIV was transmitted was never discovered. In the UK and in other countries in the developing world, there have been a number of look-back exercises involving patients that had received treatment from dentists subsequently found to be HIV-positive. None of these exercises has ever shown HIV transmission from the clinician to the patient as a result of dental treatment. During the intervening years, protocols for infection control have been significantly upgraded and enforced, thereby increasing protection of the public. The infectivity of patients living with HIV and therefore the associated risk involved in treating such patients has decreased with the introduction of antiretroviral treatment. In 1991, the Centre for Disease Control in Atlanta, USA, announced that mandatory testing and restriction of work procedures were not recommended for HIV-positive health care workers, provided they adhered to standard precautions for infection control and used safety equipment and needles (see Chapter 5). This relaxation of the regulations has not resulted in any new cases. It is hoped that this recommendation will be adopted in the UK in the future with the provision that those working in health care recognise HIV transmission in the dental care setting continues to be of concern.

HEALTH CLEARANCE FOR REGISTRATION WITH THE GENERAL DENTAL COUNCIL

The General Dental Council (GDC) health clearance requirements for dentists and dental care professional admittance to the register are shown in Box 3.1. Dentists or other dental health care personnel currently registered with the GDC who believe that they may have been exposed to blood-borne viruses are under a legal, professional and ethical obligation to promptly seek and follow confidential advice on testing for BBV and national guidelines on practising restrictions. Failure to do so may breach the duty of care to patients under the Health and Safety at Work Act and the COSHH (Control of Substances Hazardous to Health) regulations and the conditions of registration with the GDC.

Anti-discrimination legislation

Fear over the consequences of becoming HIV- or BBV-positive made someone in the profession reluctant to treat such patients in primary dental care and to refer patients to the hospital sector for treatment. Patients who have contracted HIV, HBV or HCV are entitled to receive dental treatment. Their rights are protected in the GDC's *Standards for Dental Professional*: 'Do not discriminate against patients or groups of patients because of their sex, age, race, ethnic origin, nationality, special needs or disability, sexuality, health, lifestyle, beliefs or other

> **Box 3.1** Completion of GDC health certificate as part of the procedure for registration and restoration of name for dentists and dental care professionals
>
> - Must be immunised against both hepatitis B and TB prior to obtaining health certificate
> - Must provide original evidence or certificates of immunisation
> - Dental nurses and dental technicians who do not have any clinical contact with patients must complete a self-declaration, confirming that they do not work in a clinical environment
> - All applicants who have clinical contact with patients have to submit a health certificate completed by a referee (medical practitioner or employing dentist)
>
> *Referee should assess or order additional confirmatory tests*
>
> General medical practitioner required to:
>
> - Test for immunity to hepatitis B or confirm validity of recent test
> - Confirm immunity to TB or carry out appropriate tests
> - Assess if clinical work inherently surgical involving EPP or close clinical proximity with patients
> - Assess fitness to practice, judgement and self-awareness to work professionally
> - GDP can complete the health certificate if DCP has worked in the practice >12 months; GDP has seen the original certificates of immunisation and agrees to provide an opinion

GDP, general dental practitioner; DCP, dental care professional.

irrelevant consideration'. Anti-discrimination provisions are also to be found in the Disability Discrimination Act 2005 and apply to patients with chronic disabling conditions such as HIV or cancer. The law states that a dentist should not refuse to register, or continue treating patients because of their disability.

REFERENCES AND WEBSITES

Department of Health (2007). Health clearance for tuberculosis, hepatitis B, hepatitis C and HIV: New healthcare workers. Available at http://www.dh.gov.uk, enter 'health clearance' in search box.

Salisbury, D., Ramsay, M. and Noakes, K. (2006). *Immunisation Against Infectious Disease*, 3rd edn. England: The Stationary Office, Department of Health. Available at http://www.tsoshop.co.uk or www.dh.gov.uk.

Chapter 4

Sharp safe working in the dental surgery

WHY SHARPS PREVENTION IS IMPORTANT

Sharps injuries and splashes to eyes or broken skin can transmit BBV infections.

A sharps injury refers to any injury or puncture to the skin involving a sharp instrument, e.g. dental bur, syringe needle or suture needle. Percutaneous injuries (including human bites) often produce only a minor injury to the skin, but they are clinically significant as they can transmit blood-borne viruses (BBVs), namely hepatitis C (HCV), hepatitis B (HBV) and human immunodeficiency virus (HIV). BBV can enter the tissues and cause infection following splashes into the eye, oral mucosa or on broken skin (abrasions, cuts, eczema, etc.); although the risk of transmission by these routes is considerably lower than for sharps injuries. Intact skin forms a barrier to BBV transmission and infection does not occur through inhalation or via the faecal–oral route.

In the dental surgery, the commonest route for transmission of a BBV infection is from an infected patient to a clinician. An infectious dental patient may not necessarily be identified from his or her medical history if he or she is an asymptomatic carrier. Such people are often blissfully unaware of their condition.

Considerably, less often a BBV-infected health care worker will infect a patient, or very rarely transmission occurs from patient to patient via contaminated instruments or environmental surfaces (Redd *et al.*, 2007). Look-back investigations of these outbreaks revealed that transmission tended to occur when the source person was highly contagious due to the magnitude of the viral titre in his or her bloodstream coupled with a breakdown in standard precautions. A dramatic illustration of this type of scenario is an outbreak of hepatitis B centred on an HBe antigen-positive dentist who continued working. He infected 6.9% of the patients attending his practice. Patients were infected only at the times when he omitted to wear gloves during dental treatment (Hadler *et al.*, 1981). Fortunately, occupational acquisition of HBV has declined dramatically over the past two decades because of the introduction of hepatitis B vaccination and increased adherence to standard infection control precautions.

Across the Western Europe, the prevalence of BBV in the general population is low. In the UK, 0.5–1% of the population are seropositive for HCV, approximately 0.6% for HIV and 0.1% for HBV. Although these figures can be up to ten times higher in large inner cities. The implication of these statistics is that most dental practices will have a small number of BBV seropositive patients. Following a single percutaneous injury, especially deep penetrating injuries involving a hollow-bore needle or a device visibly contaminated with blood for the probability of seroconverting is estimated at:

- 1 in 3 for HBV

- 1 in 30–50 for HCV

- 1 in 300 for HIV

- ≤1 in a 1000 for HIV for mucocutaneous (mucous membranes and skin) splashing

An alternative way of looking at these figures is that hepatitis B is 100 times and hepatitis C is 80 times more likely to be transmitted than HIV in the dental setting.

The actual risk of seroconversion is dependent on:

- Prevalence of the infection in the local population

- How infectious is the patient (i.e. high or low viral load in the blood)

- Whether the dental treatment or task is likely to result in a sharps injury

Overall, because of the low prevalence rates of BBV infections in the UK, the risk to dental staff or students of acquiring a BBV occupationally is small.

Health Protection Agency, England, conducted a survey of BBV seroconversion rates in health service staff following occupational sharps injuries from 1997 to 2005. During the 8 years of the survey, only five proven cases of occupationally acquired HIV infection (rate 0.48%) were identified (Health Protection Agency Centre for Infections, 2006). During the same period, 11 (rate 1.8%) health care personnel seroconverted to HCV, one of whom was a dentist. Doctors and dentists suffered from a disproportionately higher number of the percutaneous injuries in comparison to nurses (Health Protection Agency Centre for Infections, 2006). Worryingly, nearly 50% of the incidents were preventable. So, you cannot afford to be complacent in the way you work because of the serious and sometimes life-threatening consequences of a BBV infection (see Chapter 3). As a matter of routine, you should regard blood and blood-tainted body fluids, e.g. saliva as potentially infectious. Protect yourself and prevent onward transmission to others by applying standard precautions, wearing personnel protective equipment (PPE) and practising sharp safe working. The methods of preventing mucocutaneous exposures are discussed in Chapter 5.

WHEN DO SHARPS INJURIES OCCUR

Half of the sharps injuries are preventable.

Surveys evaluating sharps injuries affecting American and Scottish dental practitioners found that on an average they sustained 1.7–3.5 sharps injuries per year. We know that many staff are reluctant to report sharps injuries, so these figures may be an underestimate of the true number of incidents. In the Scottish study, 30% of the dentist's injuries constituted a significant exposure (i.e. source patient, HIV, HBV, HCV seropositive). A small proportion of documented injuries involve the use of increased force, bending needles or passing of sharp instruments between the dentist and the nurse. Whereas most intraoral needlestick and sharps injuries occur accidentally during the course of routine treatment as a result of sudden unexpected patient movements, closing the mouth, or as a consequence of poor visibility, such incidents are intrinsic to working in confines of the mouth. While they can be reduced to a degree by training, behavioural changes and engineering innovations, they cannot be completely eliminated.

PREVENTABLE SHARPS INJURIES

Never leave unsheathed needles on the bracket table.

Most sharps injuries happen outside the mouth, during resheathing, dismantling or disposal of needles. Such needle-stick injuries are considered 'avoidable' with safe practice. Preventive measures, e.g. safety syringes with retractable sheaves, needle guards or single-handed resheathing techniques, will significantly reduce extraoral injuries. 'Sharpless surgical techniques' that use electric scalpels, glues and clips are advocated as a safer alternative to sutures and scalpels.

Clearing up instruments at the end of treatment and manual cleaning are fraught with opportunities for sharps injuries unless precautions are taken. It is during these activities that dental nurses are most at risk. Injuries are usually sustained by the non-dominant hand. Forty per cent of extraoral injuries involve dental burs and probe tips. Fortunately, these instruments are usually less heavily contaminated with blood than hollow-bore needles and so pose less of a risk for transmission of infection. Employers are required to protect their staff from exposure to sharps injuries and BBV under the UK law as specified in the Health Care Act 2006 and COSHH (Control of Substances Hazardous to Health) regulations.

HOW TO AVOID HAVING A SHARPS INJURY

Safe disposal of needles (and scalpels) is the responsibility of the clinician.

Safe handling of sharps and needles

Injuries associated with handling and disposal of sharps and clinical waste can be minimised by adhering to accepted best practice.

Best practice guide: sharp safe dental treatment

- Use an instrument (mirror/cheek retractor) rather than fingers to retract tongue and cheeks when using sharp implements. This has the added advantage of enhancing visibility

- Do not bend the needle (as this makes resheathing difficult and is more likely to lead to injury) (Figure 4.1)

- If giving multiple injections with the same needle, recap between use

- Recap needles only using a single-handed technique or a needle guard

- Avoid passing sharp instruments from hand to hand during dental treatment

  - The same sharp instrument should not be touched by more than one person at the same time. Place the sharp in a neutral zone in the tray or bracket table from where it can safely be picked up by the second person. Alert the other person that you are putting a sharp instrument into the neutral zone.

SHARP SAFE WORKING IN THE DENTAL SURGERY

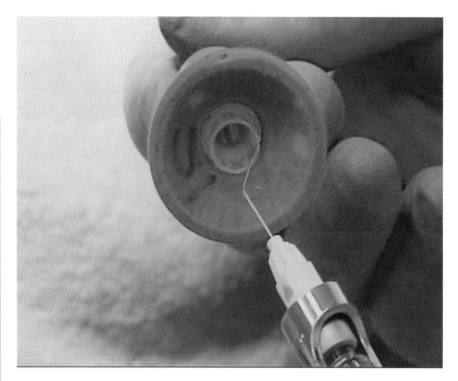

Figure 4.1 Illustration to show the difficulty in removing a bent needle with safety needle guard.

USE OF SAFETY DEVICES

Safe methods for resheathing syringe needles

> *Never resheath needles manually; use a resheathing device.*

Dentistry is unique in its continuing deployment of reusable metal syringes rather than plastic disposable syringes. They are potentially dangerous devices as resheathing and needle disassembly is undertaken at a time when the needle is contaminated with blood. Recent innovations in the design of syringes and other sharps aim to minimise both clinical and 'downstream' injuries associated with cleaning and disposing of sharps that affect nurses and cleaners.

- *Needle guards and resheathing blocks* – help to protect the hand that is used to recap the needle (Figure 4.1)

- *Safety needles with integrated retractable sheath* – the sheath can be retracted whenever the needle is required to give an injection and is then slid down over

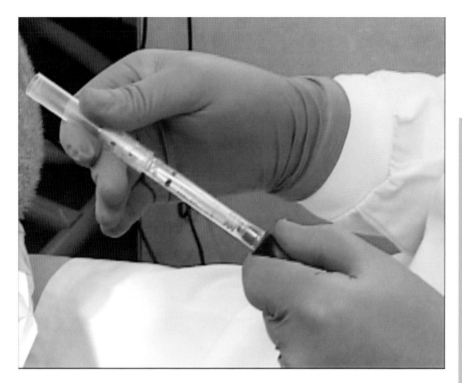

Figure 4.2 Safety needle with retractable sheath.

the needle protecting the operator between use and during dismantling and disposal (Figure 4.2). Some syringe and needle devices of the manufacturers are fully disposable as a single unit, which minimises the degree of handling

- *Needle remover on a sharps receptacle*

Best practice guide: safe resheathing of needles

- Never resheath needles manually; use a resheathing device (e.g. single-handed resheathing block, needle guard or safety needle with integrated retractable sheath)
- If a device is not readily accessible, use the 'single-handed scoop method', whereby the barrel of the syringe is held in one hand and the needle cap is scooped from a smooth hard surface onto the needle (Figure 4.3(a)). Once covered, the needle cap can be secured in place (Figure 4.3(b))

A review of needle-stick injuries across the health service in Scotland suggested that 56% of injuries would 'probably' or 'definitely' have been prevented if a safety device had been used (Young *et al.*, 2007). At a dental school in London,

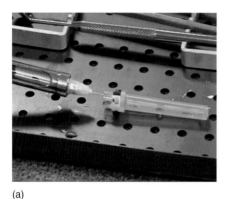

(a)

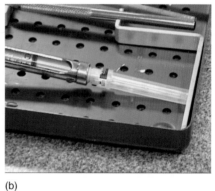

(b)

Figure 4.3 Single-handed scoop method: (a) insert needle into sheath and (b) use a firm surface to push sheath over the needle hub.

following an introductory training course in the use of the safety syringes, the number of avoidable needle-stick injuries sustained by dental students fell from 11.8 injuries/million hours worked/year down to zero (Zakrzewska *et al.*, 2001).

HOW TO AVOID SHARPS INJURIES – SHARP SAFE DISPOSAL

Best practice guide: safe disposal of sharps and needles

- Single-use sharps should be discarded immediately after use by the user
- *Never* leave sharps on the bracket table to be disposed of by someone else as this is when accidents occur
- Use disposal scalpels, which avoids the need to release the blade (Figure 4.4)
- Do not leave burs in the handpiece at the end of treatment as they can catch on skin and clothing. Remove them immediately after finishing use and then the handpiece can be dismantled from the connector and cleaned without the risk of injury
- Place disposable sharps directly into a UN-approved rigid puncture-proof sharps bin that conforms with the British Standard BS 7320 (see Chapter 10)

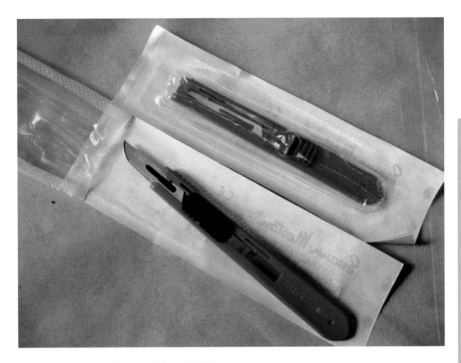

Figure 4.4 Disposable retractable scalpel blade.

SHARP SAFE WORKING IN THE DENTAL SURGERY

- When using a disposable syringe and needle discard as one unit directly into a sharps bin
- Dispose of sharps that are contaminated with saliva or blood as hazardous infectious waste in either yellow- or orange-lidded waste (Figure 4.5)

Best practice guide: assembly and use of sharps (bins) receptacles

- Ensure that the sharps bin is correctly assembled and that the lid is securely fastened before commencing use
- Place bins conveniently close to the point of use
- Do not place sharps bins on the floor, on an unstable surface or above shoulder height. They should be inaccessible to children and unauthorised persons
- Can use wall and trolley brackets to ensure that sharps bins are conveniently and securely located, especially in areas where space is limited
- Keep the aperture closed when the sharps bin is not in use

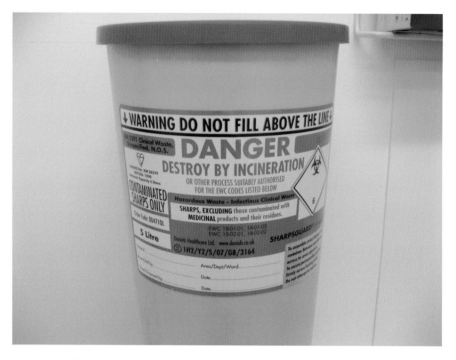

Figure 4.5 Sharps container with distinctive orange lid.

- Seal and dispose of when three-quarters full (Do not attempt to press down on contents to make more room!)
- Never try to retrieve any items from a sharps bin
- Never place sharps bins into yellow bags prior to disposal
- Always label bins with practice name, address, date and the European waste code, before disposal as hazardous waste (see Chapter 10)
- Ensure that sealed sharps bins awaiting collection are housed in a locked area, which is inaccessible to unauthorised persons

MANAGING SHARPS INJURIES

It is a requirement under the Healthcare Act 2006 that all health care workers should have access to immediate, 24-hour management of sharps injuries. Occupational injury assessment is provided either by the local occupational health department or, if this service is unavailable, by the nearest Accident and

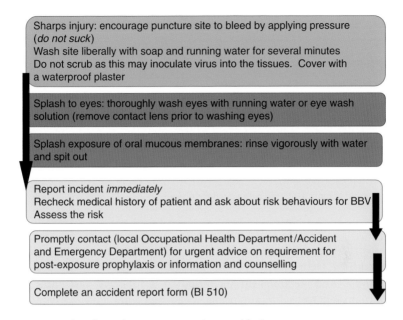

Figure 4.6 Immediate first aid: reporting procedures and further management.

Emergency Department. In order to avoid unnecessary delays the telephone number and the name of the appropriate contact person should be made known to all the staff working at the practice. Under the COSHH regulations, employers must ensure that all their staff are aware of the action to be taken following a sharps or splash incident. This includes immediate first aid, reporting procedures and further management (Figure 4.6).

OCCUPATIONAL HEALTH RISK ASSESSMENT FOR BBV EXPOSURE

Initial assessment of the injury will include whether the injury involved an accident with a sharp used on a known patient or unknown source (e.g. pooled instruments from several patients). If the source patient is known, then further information regarding the patient's risk behaviours for BBV and past medical history should be sought. The patient's responses to the questions outlined in Table 4.1 should be recorded in the 'accident' logbook.

To ensure the patient's cooperation, it is important that a staff member (preferably not the exposed person) should explain about the incident and why the additional enquiries and blood tests are being sought. The patient should be assured that strict confidentiality will be maintained throughout the process and that identifier codes rather than names can be used on the HIV test request forms.

Table 4.1 Assessment of patient's risk factors for BBV exposure

- Has the patient ever had HCV, HBV or HIV infection?
- Engaged in unprotected sex between men?
- Shared injecting equipment when using recreational drugs?
- Had unprotected sex in a country or with a person from a country where heterosexual transmission is common, e.g. Africa/Southeast Asia?
- Received a blood transfusion in the UK before 1991 or in a country where heterosexual transmission of HIV through sexual intercourse is common?
- Unprotected sexual intercourse with any of the above?

Arrange through the Occupational Health Department or hospital's Accident and Emergency Department for the patient to receive a pretest discussion (occupational and personal implications of a positive test) and to give informed consent for a blood sample to be taken for HIV, HBV and HCV testing.

How the incident is assessed and subsequently managed will be modified according to the immune status of the recipient, and if the exposure was significant (with the potential to transmit BBV). Individual responses will inform the decision on whether or not to administer HIV prophylaxis and/or a booster immunisation of hepatitis B or immunoglobulin (see Box 4.1). Following a significant exposure, a baseline and 6 months' blood samples are taken from the health care worker to establish that transmission of infection has not occurred. Blood samples are retained for 2 years.

MANAGEMENT OF HEPATITIS C EXPOSURES

At the present time there is no effective prophylaxis or vaccine available against hepatitis C. Most sharps exposures are likely to involve patients who are carriers of the disease as up to 85% of HCV infections are asymptomatic. Only HCV RNA-positive patients pose a risk for HCV transmission.

Department of Health Protocol for hepatitis C testing of health care personnel exposed to a known HCV-positive source is as follows (Health Protection Agency Centre for Infections, 2006):

- Initial baseline antibody test to HCV (to determine if the health care worker is an existing carrier of HCV)
- Obtain serum/EDTA for genome1 detection at 6 and 12 weeks

Box 4.1 Information required to assess the exposure risk to BBVs

Health care personnel's immune status for hepatitis B

- Post-vaccination hepatitis Bs-antibody titre:
  - Good responders anti-HBs level of >100 mIU/mL
  - Poor responders anti-HBs level of >10 mIU/mL but <100 mIU/mL
  - Non-responders anti-HBs level of <10 mIU/mL
- Date of administration of hepatitis B vaccination or booster inoculation

Assessment of injury: factors that increase risk of transmission of BBV

- Percutaneous needle-stick injury > mucocutaneous exposure (broken skin, abrasions, cuts, eczema etc.) or exposure of mucous membrane including the eye (splash)
- Visible blood on the device that caused the injury
- Source blood containing a high viral load

Risks associated with HIV transmission

- A deep injury
- Needle placed directly in an artery or vein
- Exposure to large volumes of blood
- A detectable viral load in a source patient currently on Highly Active Antiretroviral Treatment or terminal HIV-related illness

- Obtain serum for anti-HCV antibodies at 12 and 24 weeks
- If antibody-positive then a confirmatory HCV RNA detection test (polymerase chain reaction) is performed
- If the individual is going to receive antiviral treatment, then genotyping, viral load estimate and LFTs are undertaken

If the source of the blood is unknown then antibody levels are retested at 6 months, which allows time for viral incubation and antibody formation to occur. The subsequent results will inform the decision on whether or not to commence antiviral treatment. There is usually no need to stop performing invasive dental procedures whilst waiting for the test results. Epidemiological surveys have shown that risk of transmission of infection from a health care worker to a patient during an invasive procedure is small if standard precautions are followed.

POST-EXPOSURE PROPHYLAXIS

After the injury there is a time lag before BBV systemic spread takes place, leaving a 'window of opportunity' for HIV post-exposure prophylaxis (PEP) or stimulation of the protective immune response to hepatitis B (with a vaccine or immunoglobulin). In the UK, HIV PEP is prescribed based on a case-by-case risk assessment undertaken by the physician in conjunction with the wishes of the staff member. PEP will not normally be offered if the source case is HIV-negative or following a risk assessment that indicates the risk of HIV infection is unlikely. Note that blood from an HIV-positive source coming into contact with intact skin is not a transmission risk. In some countries, HIV PEP is offered after all occupational percutaneous exposure injuries and mucosal exposures to blood when the HIV status of the source is positive or unknown.

Antiretroviral PEP blocks replication of the initial HIV inoculum and prevents establishment of chronic HIV infection. To achieve optimal efficiency with HIV PEP, it should be started within 1 hour. This recommendation is supported by a case–control study conducted by the US Centers for Disease Control. Administration of zidovudine prophylaxis to health care personnel following occupational exposure to HIV reduced the chance of acquiring infection by 80% (Young et al., 2007). However, current guidance indicates that prophylaxis may still be of some benefit up to 2 weeks post-exposure (Young et al., 2007). Due to the success of combination therapies (HAART) in treating HIV-infected individuals, a combination of antiretroviral drugs is considered more potent than monotherapy and therefore two to four antiretroviral drugs are used for PEP.

A typical PEP regimen is shown below. Variations to this regimen may be in force locally and drug combinations may be adapted to take into account antiretroviral drug resistance in the source patient.

Department of Health, England, HIV PEP emergency starter pack:

- Travuda (300 mg tenofovir and 200 mg emtricitabine) plus
- Two Kaletra film-coated tablets (200 mg lopinavir + 50 mg ritonavir) b.d.

A full course of treatment lasts for 4 weeks, but it can be stopped if the patient is found to be HIV-negative on blood tests. Unfortunately, antiretroviral drugs cause a variety of unwanted side effects (nausea, diarrhoea, fatigue, headache etc.) as well as more serious reactions (dangerous drug interactions, diabetic exacerbation, nephrolithiasis etc.). Physicians prescribing the drugs would normally recommend strategies for managing these symptoms as it is highly desirable that the full course of treatment is completed. Over the following

---

Box 4.2 HBV post-exposure prophylaxis

- *Hepatitis B vaccine* is highly effective at preventing infection if given shortly after exposure
- Ideally, immunisation should commence within 48 hours, although it should still be considered up to a week after exposure
- The vaccine is not effective in patients with acute hepatitis B and is not necessary for individuals known to have markers of current (HBsAg) or past (anti-HB) infection. However, immunisation should not be delayed during any test results

Specific hepatitis B immunoglobulin (HBIG)

- Use of HBIG *in addition* to hepatitis B vaccine is recommended only in high-risk situations or in a known non-responder to hepatitis B vaccine
- Gives *immediate but temporary protection* after accidental inoculation or contamination with hepatitis B-infected blood. It will not affect the development of vaccine induced long-term active immunity
- HBIG is given concurrently with hepatitis B vaccine but at a different site
- Ideally, HBIG should be given within 48 hours
- HBIG should be considered up to a week after exposure as although virus multiplication may not be completely inhibited at this stage, it may prevent severe illness and development of the carrier state

---

SHARP SAFE WORKING IN THE DENTAL SURGERY

6 months, the person is monitored for symptoms of a seroconversion illness. PEP to prevent hepatitis B infection is outlined in Box 4.2.

If the student or dental personnel do become infected with HIV, hepatitis B or C, then they will need to seek specialist occupational advice as they may be prohibited from providing exposure-prone dental treatment in accordance with national guidelines (see Chapter 3).

RECORDING OF SHARPS INJURIES

All sharps injuries and significant splashes, however minor, must be recorded in an 'accident logbook'. Include a description of the accident: who was involved (both patient and staff member) and how it was managed. Data protection regulations require that the confidentiality is maintained and the information stored securely (e.g. in a lockable drawer) and retained for a minimum of 3 years. Therefore, accidents must be recorded on separate forms marked with an identification system for a chronological record keeping. Accident records may be required for future insurance or benefits claims and provide a contemporaneous evidence of a specific occupational exposure. In the UK in the event of a significant occupational exposure to HIV infection or hepatitis B or C, you may have to report the incident to Health and Safety Executive under the Reporting of Injuries, Diseases and Dangerous Occurrences (RIDDOR) Regulations. Incidents are reported either as a 'dangerous occurrence' or if HIV infection occurred then as a 'disease' (see Chapter 3). BBVs are notifiable infections in the majority of countries in the European Union. Data are collated for epidemiological purposes to facilitate contact tracing and to introduce measures to prevent onward spread of infection in the population.

CLINICAL GOVERNANCE AND ACCIDENT RISK ASSESSMENT

Reviewing clinical procedures for preventing sharps injuries and undertaking risk assessments is an important component of clinical governance and a requirement of the COSHH regulations. So, do not waste accidents and near misses; use them for staff training. It is important that the dentist creates an environment where his or her team members feel confident to inform them that something might or has gone wrong. The circumstances that lead up to the incident should be identified and analysed and appropriate steps be taken to prevent a future recurrence.

REFERENCES AND WEBSITES

Redd, J.T., Baumbach, J., Kohn, W., Nainan, O., Khristova, M. and Williams, I. (2007). Patient-to-patient transmission of hepatitis B virus associated with oral surgery. *Journal of Infectious Diseases*, 195, 1311–1314.

Hadler, S.C., Sorley, D.L., Acree, K.H. *et al.* (1981). An outbreak of hepatitis B in a dental practice. *Annals of Internal Medicine*, 95, 133–138.

Health Protection Agency Centre for Infections, National Public Health Service for Wales, CDSC Northern Ireland and Health Protection Scotland (2008). *Eye of the Needle. Surveillance of Significant Occupational Exposure to Blood borne Viruses in Healthcare Workers*. England: The Health Protection Agency. Available at http://www.hpa.org.uk/infections/topics_az/bbv/bbmenu.htm.

Young, T.N., Arens, F.J., Kennedy, G.E., Laurie, J.W. and Rutherford, G.W. (2007). Antiretroviral post-exposure prophylaxis (PEP) for occupational HIV exposure. *Cochrane Database of Systematic Reviews* 2007, Issue 1. Art. No.: CD002835. DOI: 10.1002/14651858.CD002835.pub3.

Zakrzewska, J.M., Greenwood, I. and Jackson, J. (2001). Introducing safety syringes into a UK dental school – a controlled study. *British Dental Journal*, 190, 88–92.

Further reading

Clinical Guidelines 2. Infection control. Prevention of healthcare-associated infections in primary and community care. National Institute for Clinical Excellence (NICE) (2003). Available at http://www.nice.gov.uk.

HIV Infected Health Care Workers: Guidance on Management and Patient Notification. Department of Health, England and Wales. July 2005. Available at http://www.doh.gov.uk.

Salisbury, D., Ramsay, M. and Noakes, K. (2006). *Immunisation Against Infectious Disease*, 3rd edn. Department of Health. Available at http://www.tsoshop.co.uk.

SHARP SAFE WORKING IN THE DENTAL SURGERY

Chapter 5
Hand hygiene

Microbial colonisation of the hands

The entire surface of the human body is colonised by microorganisms. High bacterial counts in the region of million colony forming bacteria per millilitre are found on the skin below the waist particularly in the warm moist perineal and inguinal areas. Lower numbers of bacteria colonise the skin of the hands, trunk and underarms. Skin colonisation increases dramatically in chronic skin conditions, e.g. dermatitis or acne. Most people shed about a million skin scales (squames) per day. Attached to the shed skin scales are microorganisms, mainly desiccation-resistant species such as staphylococci and enterococci. The shed bacteria are deposited on clothes, uniforms, masks and in the surrounding local environment.

Resident and transient bacteria

Skin of the hands harbours two main types of microorganisms, resident and transient, that colonise and survive on the hands for differing amounts of time. Resident microorganisms, as their name suggests, make up the persistent microbial flora of the hands living on the surface and within the superficial structures of the skin without causing infection. For most of the time, the bacterial relationship with the host is symbiotic. However, if the intact skin is breached by surgical interventions such as suturing then resident species (e.g. *Staphylococcus epidermidis*) can become opportunistic pathogens causing wound or deep-seated infections, whereas transient microorganisms that include environmental and pathogenic bacteria, fungi or viruses colonise the skin for short periods of time, usually only hours or days.

Following even brief episodes of personal contact, shaking hands or touching a patient's face, 100–1000 bacteria are transferred onto the dental health care personnel's hands. Not surprisingly, even higher rates of bacterial transfer can occur during patient treatment, as hands become progressively colonised with organisms from the respiratory tract and mouth. After the initial contamination of the skin, the rapidly dividing bacteria are transferred to previously uncontaminated parts of the hands, wrists or cuffs as the latter brush over the hands. Bacterial replication will continue in a linear fashion until the hands are cleaned. It is then easy to inadvertently transfer the patient's pathogenic microbes growing on the hands and inoculate your own mouth and eyes. Direct contact via hands is the major route of spread for a number of organisms including MRSA, influenza viruses and herpes viruses that cause cold sores and shingles (see Chapter 2).

HANDS AS A SOURCE OF HOSPITAL-ACQUIRED INFECTION

> Hands form a link in the chain of infection.

Hands of health care workers and patients are instrumental in the spread of multi-drug-resistant bacteria such as MRSA and *Clostridium difficile*. About 5–10% of patients during their hospital stay will pick up a healthcare associated infection (HCAI). Some of them may have fatal consequences, but all infections will add to the cost of patient treatment and cause unnecessary suffering and inconvenience to the patient and their family and friends. In the USA, 2 000 000 patients become seriously ill as a result of acquiring an infection in hospital with approximately 80 000 deaths annually. In England, healthcare associated infection costs in the region of £3–8000 per infection. Yet, this unwelcome chain of events can be broken simply and expediently by effective use of hand hygiene. Results from the data collected over the last 30 years provide strong evidence that hand hygiene is the single most important method of reducing cross-transmission of infectious organisms (Pratta *et al.*, 2007).

HAND HYGIENE AND TEAMWORKING

The foundation for the World Health Organization (WHO) campaign to promote hand hygiene was the compelling results from the longitudinal study by Pittet *et al.* (2000) working in hospitals in Geneva, Switzerland. They introduced alcohol/chlorhexidine gluconate 0.5% hand rub solution as the focal point of a hospital-wide hand hygiene campaign. With the cooperation of the hospital staff their campaign achieved an impressive 44% reduction in HCAI and a 50% fall in patient colonisation with MRSA. An important lesson was learnt from their work of direct relevance to dental practice. Long-term success (the study was conducted over 6 years) was dependent on the active

HAND HYGIENE

involvement of senior personnel who were publically seen to endorse the campaign. Posters and other promotional material reinforced the main message of the campaign and staff received regular feedback from local audits evaluating their compliance with hand hygiene measures. Similarly, dentists as team leaders can influence the behaviour of other members of their team by acting as positive role models. Staff are more likely to follow suit and embrace protocols, if dentists or, in the case of dental schools, professors are witnessed to actively comply with infection control measures.

Choosing the correct hand hygiene product

The new term 'hand hygiene' encompasses traditional hand washing with soap and water or aqueous antimicrobial detergents and the newer technique of hand rubbing with alcohol-based products (gels, rinses and foams) that do not require running water.

Not all skin-cleaning agents are equally effective at removing organic material or killing microbes (see Table 5.1). So, choosing the most appropriate agent for hand hygiene will depend on when and why the hands are being cleaned. Hand hygiene is used in three circumstances: social, antiseptic and surgical (see Table 5.2). It is impossible to completely sterilise the hands as resident bacteria survive in the deep skin hair follicles and sebaceous glands, but if hands are cleaned effectively only very low numbers of bacteria will remain (see Figure 5.1).

Table 5.1 Comparison of the properties of common hand hygiene products

Type of hand-cleaning agent	Action	Inhibited by organic material	Active against *C. difficile*	Limitations	Type of hand hygiene
Chlorhexidine and triclosan	Rapid Binds to skin; remains active for up to 6 hours	No	Yes	Chlorhexidine may cause irritant dermatitis in some people	Clinical Surgical
Iodophors	Rapid	Yes	Yes	Inhibited by organic material	Surgical
Alcohol hand rubs and gels	Very rapid Short-lived	Yes	No	Inhibited by organic material	Clinical Surgical

HAND HYGIENE

Table 5.2 The three types of hand washing

Type	Product	Duration (Entire procedure)	Purpose
Social hand washing	Soap and water	20–30 seconds	Removal of dirt, body fluids and transient microorganisms
Clinical hand hygiene	Aqueous antimicrobial disinfectant	20–30 seconds	Killing and removal of transient microbes and reduction of resident flora
	Alcohol hand rub	20–30 seconds	
Surgical hand hygiene	Aqueous antimicrobial disinfectant alcohol hand rub	2 minutes	Killing and removal of transient microorganisms and substantially reduction of resident microorganisms

Alcohol hand rubs

> *Alcohol hand rubs are recommended for clinical hand hygiene by the WHO.*

Alcohol hand rubs were originally promoted by health care campaigners to encourage improved compliance and overcome perceived and real barriers to hand washing. In surveys, conventional detergents and soaps were shunned by health care personnel as being damaging to the skin. Inconveniently located sinks and time constraints were also cited as reasons not to wash hands.

Alcohol hand rubs have the advantage of containing an emollient to protect the skin, are inexpensive and hand hygiene can be performed at the chair side. Hand rubs are available in an individual dispenser that can be carried in the

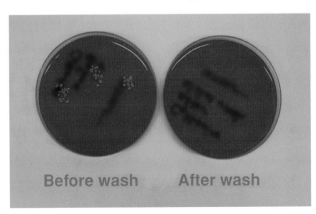

Figure 5.1 Microbiological hand sampling before and after washing with alcohol hand rub.

pocket or on a belt and are ideal where there is limited access to a sink such as on a domiciliary visit. Commercial products are diluted from 10 to 40% by weight with water to enhance denaturation of microbial proteins. Alcohols demonstrate rapid action against a wide range of Gram-positive and Gram-negative species including MRSA and vancomycin-resistant enterococcus. As little as 15 seconds of vigorous hand rubbing has been shown to be effective in preventing transmission of Gram-negative bacteria. Although most manufacturers and the WHO recommend cleaning the hands for 30 seconds, allowing the alcohol to completely evaporate from hands is essential for microbial killing (WHO, 2006).

Limitations of alcohol hand rubs

> Use alcohol hand rub only on visibly clean hands.

Alcohol-based products have limitations which need to be recognised if they are to be used safely. Although alcohol products are specifically designed to promote the frequency of hand hygiene at busy times, their deceptive ease of use can lead to tokenistic, cursory decontamination of the hands with increasing workload. They lack any detergent effect and are unsuitable when hands are heavily contaminated or are visibly soiled. Importantly, they are ineffective against spore-forming bacteria e.g. *C. difficile* or enteroviruses. Paradoxically, recent overreliance on alcohols and the concomitant reduction in traditional hand washing with soaps ands detergents may be contributing to the increasing incidence of *C. difficile* diarrhoeal infections in the UK. Unlike chlorhexidine, their action is only short-lived. The alcohol component evaporates rapidly, often before the user has been able to spread the solution over all parts of their hands, so areas escape exposure to the bactericidal action of the alcohol. Gels formulations overcome this problem by slowing down evaporation, increasing the active contact time and thereby enhancing bacterial killing. The emollient added to hand rubs and gels can build up on hands giving a feeling of greasiness which some people find distasteful. Excess emollient is also transferred from hands to clinic surfaces contaminating them. To avoid these problems, hands should be washed with plain soap and water at intervals throughout the day.

Storage of alcohol hand rub

Alcohol-based hand rub is flammable and has a low flash point and can be ignited by static electricity. Care should be taken to avoid splashing near an open flame or contact with direct heat or sunlight, especially when it is stored in bulk. Fortunately, the number of fires directly attributable to combustion of alcohol hand rub is few. As is the case with all disinfectants, a COSHH (Control of Substances Hazardous to Health) safety assessment is advised. Try to keep it out of reach of children who might be tempted to drink it! Avoiding the term 'alcohol' in signs and patient information literature will help to dissuade curious or desperate patients from taking a surreptitious swig.

When to clean your hands

Hands must be cleaned immediately *before* each and every episode of dental treatment or *after* contact with saliva, blood or other bodily fluid (see Figure 5.2). It is very easy to contaminate inanimate objects in the surgery unthinkingly by touching them with gloved hands during patient treatment. At particular risk from hand and environmental contamination are computer keyboards, pens and patient's notes. In hospital studies nearly all patients' case notes were contaminated with pathogenic bacteria, including MRSA. Reception staff and others are advised to clean hands after touching notes or surfaces in close proximity to patients.

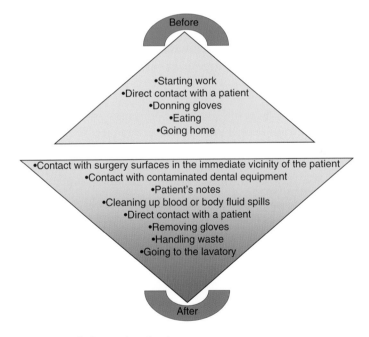

Figure 5.2 Summary of when to clean hands.

HAND HYGIENE TECHNIQUE

Remove rings and watches

Microbiological studies have shown that the skin under rings becomes heavily colonised with bacteria, e.g. *Staphylococcus aureus* and Gram-negative species.

The same bacterial species were found to persist for months under a ring. Fewer bacteria are found under silver than gold and platinum rings, as silver is inhibitory to the growth of bacteria. Rings and watches may also prevent effective cleaning of the skin because the wearer does not want to damage or loose a precious item of jewellery and avoids cleaning the hands effectively. Therefore, it is recommended that watches and rings (except for plain wedding bands) are removed before the start of the treatment session. Moreover, gloves are more prone to tear when rings are worn. Artificial nails and chipped nail polish also harbour bacteria and *Candida* spp. Artificial nails have been implicated as the source of outbreaks of bacterial and fungal infections amongst patients in hospital wards. So, it is best to keep fingernails short, clean and free from nail polish and artificial nails.

Ayliffe hand hygiene technique

The Ayliffe hand washing technique is versatile and appropriate for social, clinical and surgical hand hygiene. It can be used to apply soap, aqueous antimicrobial hand wash and alcoholic hand rub to the hands. At the start of a treatment session, hands should be washed with soap and water and thereafter alcohol hand gel can be used as long as hands remain visibly clean. There is a science to hand washing/cleaning in the same way as there is to cleaning teeth effectively. By employing a standardised method (e.g. the Ayliffe technique), this ensures that all surfaces of the hands and wrists are exposed to the disinfectant and thoroughly cleaned in a systematic manner. The sequence of hand movements is formulated to concentrate on the heavily contaminated fingertips and areas of the hand that are missed, e.g. finger and thumb webs as shown in Figure 5.3. None of the disinfectants used in antimicrobial soaps are particularly effective at killing spore-forming bacteria. It is now appreciated that

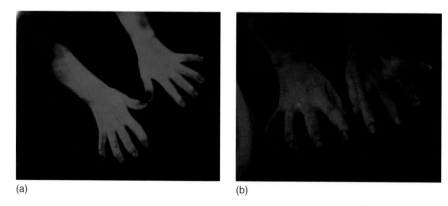

(a)   (b)

Figure 5.3 (a) UV-sensitive alcohol hand rub is applied to all parts of the hands and wrists before cleaning them. (b) After cleaning hands. *Note*: Areas of hands that are missed still glow under the UV light.

HAND HYGIENE

removal of spores from the hands requires the physical action of vigorous rubbing and rinsing under running water. The final stage is thoroughly drying the hands. This helps to maintain skin integrity and prevent onward transmission of microbes, which can proliferate on damp hands and damaged skin. Moist hands transfer a significantly larger number of microbes to hard surfaces and fabrics than hands that are carefully dried.

When using the Ayliffe technique (Figure 5.4) with alcohol solutions, it is important to use a sufficient quantity of hand gel/rub to thoroughly cover all

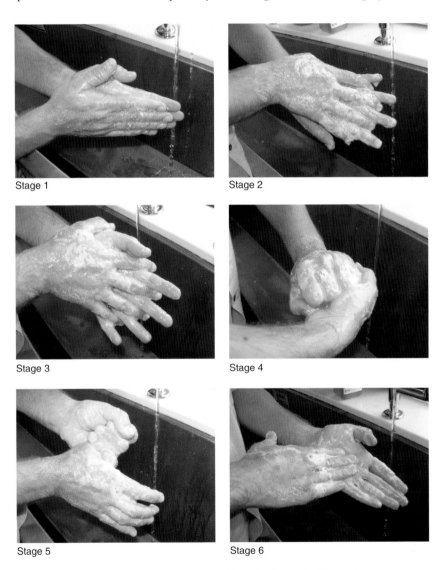

Figure 5.4 The Ayliffe hand hygiene technique. (Photos kindly supplied by Paul Morris, Queen's University Belfast.)

surfaces of the hands. Recently, the WHO has recommended that the cupped palm of the hand is completely filled with hand rub solution (approximately 3–5 mL) in order to achieve total hand coverage before vigorous hand rubbing for 30 seconds.

Best practice guide: preparation for hand hygiene

- A poster showing hand washing protocol should be displayed in the surgery
- Cuts and abrasions <24 hours old must be covered with a waterproof dressing. After 24 hours, the body's natural defences 'seal' small cuts and wounds
- Fingernails should be kept short, clean and free from nail polish, artificial nails and nail art
- Wrist watches and jewellery should be removed, and long-sleeved clothing be rolled up/removed. Rings (except wedding rings) should not be worn during a clinical session. Manipulate wedding ring when washing hands so that cleaning solution can contact skin under the ring
- Hand cream should be applied regularly throughout the day to protect skin from drying. However, communal tubs should be avoided as these can become contaminated

Hand hygiene technique: social and antiseptic hand washing

Hand washing with liquid soap or aqueous antimicrobial hand wash solutions:

- Washing procedure take 20–30 seconds
- Wet hands under lukewarm running water before applying liquid soap or antiseptic hand wash solution into cupped hands. Use enough soap/antiseptic solution to cover the hands completely
- Rub hands together vigorously to lather all surfaces of hands and wrists
- Wash palms, backs of hands, finger and thumb webs, tips of fingers and thumbs, especially the nail area (see Figure 5.4)
- Rinse hands thoroughly under running water
- Dry hands completely with a soft, absorbent single-use disposable paper towel
- Use the disposable towel to turn off the tap

HAND HYGIENE

Hand hygiene using an alcohol hand rub/gel

- Fill a cupped hand with alcohol gel solution

- Distribute alcohol hand rub solution evenly over every part of the hand, fingers and wrists

- Rub hands together vigorously using the Ayliffe method for 20–30 seconds. Pay particular attention to the tip webs and nail beds of the fingers and thumbs

- Continue until the solution has completely evaporated and the hands are dry

Surgical hand washing

For surgical procedures (e.g. implant surgery), more extensive disinfection of the hands (antisepsis) is required in order to reduce the numbers of resident bacteria to a minimum, although it is not possible to sterilise the skin. First, clean the nails and then wash the hands and forearms with an antimicrobial disinfectant hand wash solution for 2 minutes, followed by thorough rinsing and drying of the skin.

Alternatively, use an alcohol hand rub. Prewash hands and forearms with a mild neutral soap and water and clean nails followed by two sequential 5-mL applications of alcohol hand rub gel. Vigorously rub hands and forearms using the standard method described above until completely dry. Comparative experiments have shown that the two-stage technique with alcohol hand rubs is as effective as conventional hand scrubbing with an antimicrobial-disinfectant hand wash solution. Using either method the bacterial counts will remain sufficiently low throughout a 4-hour surgical procedure.

HAND CARE AND PREVENTION OF IRRITANT DERMATITIS

The keratin-rich layers of intact skin form a natural barrier to infection, so it is essential that you protect your hands from damage by wearing heavy duty gloves for work in the home and garden. Sebum from the sebaceous glands helps to maintain skin integrity. Skin pH is mildly acidic. Regular use of alkaline soaps and disinfectants can alter the pH and cause drying and abrasion of the hands, which in some people can result in irritant dermatitis. Alcohols are inherently drying. Products containing 70% alcohol by weight cause the least dehydration of the skin and are the most popular with users. To compensate for the dehydrating effect, manufacturers add emollients, which is why these products cause less abrasions, drying and irritation to the hands than soaps or disinfectants.

HAND HYGIENE

Staff members or students who have an existing skin condition such as dermatitis or who develop skin irritation whilst using particular products such as gloves or disinfectants should seek expert advice on treatment and management. Allergenicity is routinely reported with antimicrobial detergent solutions; the latter may also cause drying and abrasion of the skin on repeated use, whereas alcohol has a low allergenic potential. However, as may occur with any skin preparation, a small proportion of people do develop hypersensitivity to alcohol-based hand rubs. Allergic reactions and cases of contact dermatitis are usually in response to the other added ingredients. Affected health care personnel should change to an alternative product and seek medical advice from their local occupational health physician or general medical practitioner.

Protective effect of emollient hand creams

Emollient hand cream applied several times a day help to prevent skin problems from developing. Shared communal pots of hand cream become rapidly contaminated, so either individual supplies or elbow-operated pump dispensers of hand cream are advised. Petroleum-based hand creams are not recommended as they can adversely affect latex, thereby increasing glove permeability, which in turn permits ingress of microorganisms. Furthermore, hand cream has been demonstrated to reduce cross-transmission by preventing excess shedding of residential bacteria from dry, flaky skin.

Best practice guide: consumables and facilities for hand hygiene area

- Sink, taps and tile surrounds should be visibly clean and free of clutter

- Easily accessible dedicated hand washing sink with no overflows or plugs; and mixer taps to avoid scalding

- To reduce formation of contaminated aerosol basins, the water jet should not flow directly into the plughole

- Taps should preferably be microprocessor, elbow-, wrist- or foot-operated taps to reduce the risk of hand contamination

- A choice of wall-mounted dispensers of liquid soap, aqueous detergent and alcohol hand rub should be provided

- Hand hygiene solutions should be dispensed in disposable rather than refillable cartridges/bottles. Refillable dispensers, which become contaminated with microorganisms during the 'topping up' process unless thoroughly decontaminated including the nozzle, should be avoided

- Soap bars are not suitable for use in the clinical setting as they easily become colonised with Gram-negative bacteria and *Pseudomonas* spp. and act as a source of cross-infection

HAND HYGIENE

- Wall-mounted disposable paper towels should be used. Reusable towels are not suitable for clinical settings as they become readily contaminated with microorganisms. Dispose in foot-operated waste bins. Do not use your hands to raise the lid

- Nailbrushes are *not* indicated for hand hygiene in dental practice. If nails need to be cleaned before surgery, then a sterile brush should be used on each occasion

- A wall-mounted dispenser of alcohol hand gel should be provided in patient waiting room

Patients should be encouraged to clean their hands with alcohol hand gel on entering and exiting the treatment area, as they are part of the chain of infection. This is particularly relevant when patients have been coughing or sneezing.

REFERENCES AND WEBSITES

Pittet, D., Hugonnet, S., Mourouga, P. *et al.* (2000). Effectiveness of a hospital-wide programme to improve compliance with hand hygiene. *Lancet, 356,* 1307–1312.

Pratta, R.J., Pellowea, C.M., Wilson, J.A. *et al.* (2007). Epic2: National evidence-based guidelines for preventing healthcare-associated infections in NHS Hospitals in England. *Journal of Hospital Infection, 65S,* S1–S64.

World Health Organization (2006). *WHO Guidelines on Hand Hygiene in Health Care (Advanced Draft), World Alliance for Patient Safety.* Geneva: WHO. Available at www.who.int/entity/patientsafety/events/05/HH_en.pdf.

HAND HYGIENE

Chapter 6

Personal protection for prevention of cross-infection

Personal protective equipment (PPE) such as gowns, goggles, masks and disposable gloves form a protective barrier to reduce contamination of clothing, skin and mucous membranes from patient's body fluids or splatter. The Health and Safety at Work Act 1974 and the subsequent legislation place a duty of care on employers to provide a safe working environment for their staff, provide PPE and train staff to use it appropriately. Staff and students must ensure their own safety by wearing PPE. Selection of PPE must be based on a risk assessment of the associated hazard and likelihood of transmission of microorganisms to the patient. The practice of infection control policy should reflect:

- Type and duration of the task
- Potential for exposure to blood and body fluids
- Potential for contamination of non-intact skin or mucous membranes

PPE will function effectively only if selected, worn, removed and discarded correctly. In terms of risk management and according to the law, PPE is considered a 'method of last resort' as PPE is not foolproof and only reduces rather than eliminates the risk (Table 6.1).

Under the European law, PPE is classified as a medical device. Therefore, only products carrying the European CE mark denoting that the product fulfils specified performance standards should be worn.

THE ROLE OF GLOVES

Gloves should be worn for all routine dental treatments and discarded between patients.

Table 6.1 Risk management hierarchy

Hierarchy of infection control procedures for personal protection	Examples
Elimination of the hazard	Single-use instruments
Isolation of the hazard	Safety needles
Work practice controls	Hand hygiene
Work behaviour controls	User disposes of sharps
Administrative controls	Infection control policy
Personal protective equipment	Masks, gloves, aprons

When used correctly, wearing gloves:

- Protects hands from contamination with blood, saliva and microorganisms

- Reduces the risk of cross-infection

- Protects hands from toxic and irritant chemicals

- Does not prevent sharps injuries, but the wiping effect of the glove reduces the risk of contamination

Gloves should be worn during routine dental and surgical treatment, when cleaning instruments, handling waste or mopping up spills. If they are not removed at the end of a task, they become equivalent to 'a second skin', acting as a source of infection. Acquisition and growth dynamics of microorganisms are similar on bare and gloved hands. Beware: wearing gloves can give a false sense of security to the wearer as they do not provide complete protection against hand contamination.

Best practice guide: safe use of gloves in the dental surgery

- Hands must be washed before donning gloves. Never consider gloves to be an alternative to hand washing

- Changing your gloves between patients prevents cross-transmission between patients and contamination of hard surfaces in the surgery. Do not touch patient's notes, pens, computer keyboards, door or drawer handles, or your face with gloved hands (see Chapter 8)

- *Never* reuse single-use disposable gloves. There is clinical evidence to demonstrate that glove reuse is associated with transmission of MRSA and Gram-negative bacilli

PERSONAL PROTECTION FOR PREVENTION OF CROSS-INFECTION

- Never wash single-use gloves; it reduces the barrier properties

- Keep glove wear to a minimum. Gloves should be applied immediately before starting treatment and removed as soon as the activity is complete

- Dispose of gloves as hazardous infectious waste

- Change gloves during very long procedures. After prolonged use, approximately 9–12% of gloves develop perforations or become porous due to hydration of the latex and may leak. Hepatitis viruses have been transmitted via minor glove perforations

- Changing your gloves during long procedures reduces excess sweating, which in turn decreases dermal infections or inflammation

- Remember that hands are not necessarily clean because gloves have been worn. On removing gloves, the patient's microorganisms can be transmitted from the external surface of the glove to the dentist's hands and need to be removed by hand hygiene

CHOOSING A SUITABLE GLOVE FOR THE TASK

Natural rubber latex (NRL) gloves and nitrile gloves permit good manual dexterity, are impermeable to microbes and are the commonest types of glove used or clinical procedures (see Table 6.2).

Double gloving has been recommended for high-risk surgical procedures. Using a coloured inner glove increases the user's awareness of glove perforation during surgery.

MANAGING AN ALLERGY TO NRL GLOVES

Reports on the prevalence of latex sensitivity amongst health care workers (and patients) have risen to 6–18%, paralleling the increased clinical use of latex gloves from the mid-1980s onwards. Latex sensitivity is particularly common amongst dental students and staff, and can develop even after successfully wearing NRL gloves for many years. Sensitivity occurs after inhalation of airborne latex antigens or absorption through damaged skin. NRL is a plant product, but other chemicals are added during fabrication of the glove to imbue it with strength, elasticity and flexibility. Varying amounts of NRL and chemical residues may still be present in the glove as a consequence of the manufacturing process. It is advised to wear gloves with low levels of extractable proteins

Table 6.2 Properties of examination and surgical gloves

Type of glove	Properties	Allergies
Natural rubber latex	Impermeable to BBV, close fitting, do not impair dexterity and are not prone to splitting resistance to water-based chemicals	Not suitable if allergy to NRL or accelerator
Acrylonitrile (nitrile)	Impermeable to BBV, close fitting, do not impair dexterity and are not prone to splitting (lowest failure rate under stress conditions), resistance to solvents and oil-based chemicals	Not suitable if allergy to nitrile or accelerator in NRL gloves
Polychloroprene (neoprene)	Impermeable to BBV	Suitable if allergy to NRL
Vinyl	Impermeable to BBV and has similar properties to NRL when made to the European Standard. If not, vinyl may be permeable to blood-borne viruses, rigid, inflexible and break down in use	Suitable if allergy to NRL
Copolymer (multipolymer synthetic styrene-ethylene-butadiene-styrene), e.g. Tactylon	Similar elasticity and strength to NRL	Contains no NRL proteins and chemicals and are suitable for people with NRL sensitivity
Polythene	Permeable, ill-fitting and prone to splitting and tearing, not suitable for clinical use	Not applicable

BBV, blood-borne virus; NRL, natural rubber latex.

(<50 μg/g of latex proteins) and chemical accelerators ($<0.1\%$ w/w of residual accelerators) to minimise the risk of sensitisation.

Reactions are classified as:

- *Delayed hypersensitivity* (type IV) – resulting in contact dermatitis, rhinitis and conjunctivitis. This is the most common hypersensitivity reaction to NRL or accelerating agents. Response occurs between 6 and 48 hours after exposure

- *Immediate hypersensitivity* (type I) – asthma, urticaria, laryngeal oedema and anaphylactic shock/collapse. Response occurs 15–30 minutes after exposure

Creating a low-latex or latex-free environment

The risk of allergic reactions is triggered not only by latex gloves but also by other latex-containing devices, e.g. rubber dam, syringe and medication vial

PERSONAL PROTECTION FOR
PREVENTION OF CROSS-INFECTION

bungs, prophylaxis cups, orthodontic elastics etc. In practices with sensitised individuals, all the dental team may need to change to non-latex gloves due to the generation of aeroallergens in the surgery environment. Susceptible clerical staff who do not have direct contact with the patient can also become sensitised as the latex aerosols travel on air currents permeating office areas and waiting rooms. Environmental contamination with latex proteins can be reduced by: good ventilation, regular changes of ventilation filters, extensive vacuuming and cleaning of surface contaminated with latex allergens. Equipment in the dental emergency kit should also be free from latex.

Treatment and avoidance strategies are most effective when initiated early. This relies on recognising the symptoms of immediate and delayed hypersensitivity reactions both on oneself and in patients. If latex sensitivity is suspected, the student, staff member or patient should be referred for specialist advice. Individuals who have experienced a type I reaction to NRL are strongly advised to wear a Medic Alert bracelet.

Alternative to NRL gloves that have similar physical properties, i.e. do not impair dexterity and are not prone to splitting and are impermeable to blood-borne viruses, are shown in Table 6.2. According to Health and Safety Law in the UK, staff sensitised to NRL gloves must be supplied with appropriate alternatives by their employer. In response to their medicolegal requirements, a number of dental schools and health care centres have opted to go latex-free as a prophylactic measure to prevent triggering problems in patients, students and staff.

MANAGING LATEX ALLERGIES IN PATIENTS

Patients may not always be aware that they have a latex allergy. Individuals who are atopic (predisposition to allergic reactions, e.g. hay fever, asthma and eczema) are at an increased risk of developing a hypersensitivity reaction to NRL.

Best practice guide: managing latex allergies

- The medical history includes a question on latex allergy (e.g. hypersensitivity reaction following contact with household gloves, blowing up balloons, or food allergies to banana, avocado and kiwi fruit which possess shared antigens with NRL)

- If allergy is known, ensure that dental notes are clearly labelled

- Use latex-free gloves, rubber dams and equipment

- Remind these patients to inform reception staff when making an appointment and the dentist prior to treatment

MASKS, VISORS AND GOGGLES AND THE PROTECTION OF MUCOUS MEMBRANES AND THE AIRWAY

The choice of PPE for the face is based on the likelihood of being splashed with blood or contaminated aerosols. In addition to wearing PPE, using safe working practices will help to prevent exposure of mucous membranes and non-intact skin including:

- Avoid touching the mouth, nose, eyes or face with contaminated hands or gloves

- Careful fitting of PPE before patient's contact to avoid the need to make further adjustments to the PPE during treatment

- Use of suction to reduce volume of spray and splatter

- Use of rubber dams to avoid direct exposure to patient's respiratory secretions

TYPES OF MASKS AND WHEN TO USE THEM

Surgical face masks – protecting the patient during surgery

Masks protect the wearer from splatter and aerosols.

Surgical face masks were originally developed over a century ago with the primary aim of protecting patient's open wounds from skin squames and respiratory droplets expelled by the surgeon. In England, postoperative infections are responsible for an additional 6.5 days of hospital stay per patient and doubling of hospital costs.

Recently, reassessment of the role masks play in reducing perioperative infection rates has produced equivocal findings (Lipp and Edwards, 2002). Some authors have even suggested that the design of the mask might potentially contribute to wound infections. Masks have a multi-layer construction at the centre of which are two filters, each with a 1-μm filtering efficiency capable of trapping microbes and skin squames of that size or larger. They provide protection for up to 2 hours, unless they become wet. Expired air is moist and eventually makes the mask wet. It then acts as a wick, enhancing the movement of bacteria by capillary action from the inner to the outer surface of the mask. In addition, friction from the mask rubbing against the face increases dispersal of facial skin scales and the chance of surgical wound contamination. So, wearing a traditional mask specifically to prevent surgical wound infections is questionable. Prevention of surgical wound infections is complex and depends on multiple factors that are not influenced by wearing a mask.

Masks as PPE

Masks are now advocated as a protective barrier for students and health care personnel exposed to droplet and aerosol contamination. Mucous membranes of the mouth, nose and non-intact skin surfaces compromised by acne or dermatitis are susceptible portals for infection. Masks are resistant to fluids and act as a physical barrier protecting the wearer from splashes and sprays.

Masks come in various shapes (e.g. moulded and non-moulded), filtration efficiency and method of attachment (e.g. ties, elastic and ear loops). They are disposable and intended for single use only. When worn correctly, the mask should cover the nose and mouth. If the mask is fitted with metal nose band, this is contoured to the bridge of the nose. If the tapes are not sufficiently tight then the mask will leak around the sides and become ineffective. Nevertheless, most masks produce a relatively poor facial seal, and the air is not effectively filtered on inhalation into the lungs. Hence, masks provide minimal or partial protection of the wearer from respiratory pathogens such as *Mycobacteria tuberculosis* or influenza.

Best practice guide: how to use a medical mask

- Masks are recommended for all dental procedures
- Masks should be close fitting and cover the nose and mouth (Figure 6.1)
- Touching the outer filtering surface of the mask, which may be contaminated, should be avoided
- The mask should not be removed by breaking, undoing the ties or lifting over the ears. Ties are considered 'clean' and can be touched with bare hands
- Masks are single-use items. They should be changed after every patient and not reused
- Mask should be disposed of immediately after use as hazardous clinical waste
- Hands should be cleaned after removing the mask in order to prevent contamination of your face and the surgery environment

Respiratory hygiene

The third use for medical face masks is respiratory hygiene. Lessons learnt during the SARS (severe acute respiratory syndrome) outbreak in 2003 demonstrated that infection was spread by undiagnosed patients coughing as they waited their turn for treatment in clinic waiting rooms (Seto *et al.*, 2003). It is anticipated that cough etiquette protocols would become necessary in practice

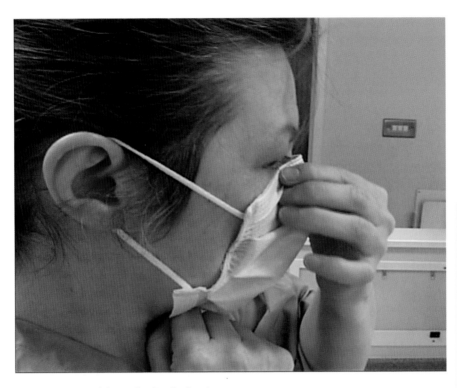

Figure 6.1 A mask being fitted to the facial contours.

waiting area during an outbreak of respiratory illness such as pandemic flu. In this situation, patients would be asked politely to wear a mask to prevent spread of infection from themselves to others. Alternatively, if patients are unwilling or unable to wear a mask, then they would be asked to cover the mouth/nose with a tissue when coughing and promptly dispose of used tissues and then clean their hands with alcohol hand rub. Ideally, patients should be seated >3 feet apart. Physical proximity of <3 feet from an infected person has been associated with increased droplet route transmission of serious infections, e.g. *Neisseria meningitidis* and group A streptococcus.

Respirator masks

> *Respirator masks are used during the care of patients with respiratory infections transmitted by airborne particles.*

Particulate respirator masks offer a higher degree of personal respiratory protection compared to a standard medical face mask. They are designed to filter out airborne particles <5 μm in size in the inspired air. Only respirators with CE markings that conform to the European Standard EN149:2001 should be

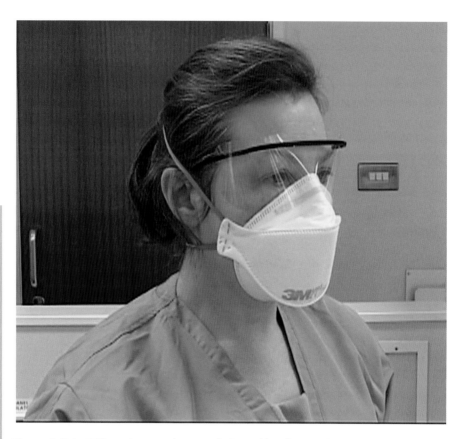

Figure 6.2 An FFP2 respirator mask worn with disposable safety goggles.

worn. The standard defines performance parameters of the respirator mask including filtration efficiency. The European Standard EN149:2001 FFP2 (94% filtering efficiency) is recommended for use when treating patients with active tuberculosis (see Figure 6.2). Particulate respirator masks are currently recommended when treating patients with diseases spread by respiratory aerosols, e.g. influenza, SARS, measles, varicella and tuberculosis. Masks with a higher filtering efficiency are recommended by the Health Protection Agency (European Standard EN149:2001 FFP3 (98% filtering efficiency)) for suspected or probable cases of avian or pandemic flu.

Respirator masks like other PPE should not be relied on for sole protection, but should be used in combination with appropriate surgery ventilation and immunisation where available. When purchasing respirator masks, select models with inherently good fit characteristics, i.e. those expected to provide protection factors of 10 or more to 95% of wearers. Some countries such as the USA recommend a comprehensive programme including fit testing of the mask, medical clearance to wear a respirator, education on respirator use and periodic re-evaluation of the respiratory protection protocol.

Best practice guide: fitting and wearing a respirator mask

- When fitted and worn correctly, respirators seal firmly to the face, thus reducing the risk of leakage

- A user seal check should be performed by the wearer of a respirator each time it is donned to minimise air leakage around the facepiece. These differ slightly with each product and are supplied by the manufacturer

- Note that beards and stubble interfere with the fit and seal of the respirator

- Avoid touching the outer surface of the respirator mask once it is fitted. Always clean hands after handling the mask

- Dispose of as hazardous clinical waste

There are no evidence-based data on which to base a recommendation for the length of time a respirator mask may be reused. Manufacturer's data sheets normally only specify the length of time filtering efficiency of the mask is guaranteed for continuous wear. Therefore continuous use of the respirator by the same individual during the same clinical session is an acceptable practice, provided the respirator is not damaged or soiled, the fit is not compromised by change in shape, and the respirator has not been contaminated with blood or body fluids.

PROTECTION DURING CARDIOPULMONARY RESUSCITATION

Mouthpieces, pocket resuscitation masks with one-way valves and other ventilation devices provide a safe alternative to mouth-to-mouth resuscitation, preventing exposure of the caregiver's nose and mouth to oral and respiratory fluids during the procedure.

PROTECTIVE EYEWEAR AND VISORS

The clinical dental team must protect their own eyes and those of the patient against splatter, aerosols and foreign bodies such as amalgam fragments. Spectacles and contact lenses are not considered adequate eye protection. Ideally, eye protection (goggles or face shields) should be comfortable and allow for sufficient peripheral vision, secure fit and offer protection from splashes, sprays and respiratory droplets from multiple angles. Many styles of goggles fit adequately over spectacles with minimal gaps. While effective as eye protection, goggles do not provide splash or spray protection to other parts of the face. Use of goggles was shown to protect the wearer from occupational infection with respiratory syncytial virus (RSV) which is spread by respiratory droplets. Whether this was due to preventing hand–eye contact or respiratory droplet–eye contact has not been determined. Goggles provide suitable protection for the eyes when splashing is likely, whilst face shields are best worn where there is a risk of blood splattering or aerosolisation of potentially infectious material as they provide full-face protection.

PROTECTIVE EYEWEAR

Best practice guide: goggles and face shields

Goggles

- Goggles or face shields should be worn during all types of dental treatment or when manually cleaning instruments

- Choose goggles with side protection that conform to standard BS EN 166:1988

- Goggles should be decontaminated according to the manufacturer's instructions, e.g. alcohol-based surface disinfectant or hypochlorite diluted to 1000 ppm available chlorine, followed by thorough rinsing in water

- In the event of contamination of the eyes with blood or other body fluids or chemicals, first remove contact lens (if worn) and then rinse the eye with copious amounts of eye wash or cold water. If the source patient is a carrier of a blood-borne virus then follow the advice for managing a sharps/splash incident outlined in Chapter 4

- Goggles should not impair the operator's vision as this could result in compromised patient care. If they become scratched or cloudy following multi-use they should be replaced

Face shields

- Spectacles do not provide sufficient eye protection, so wear a face shield over them (Figure 6.3)

- Clip-on visors can be worn over loupes and protect the eyepieces from contamination

- Visors have the added advantage of discouraging touching the face with contaminated gloved hands

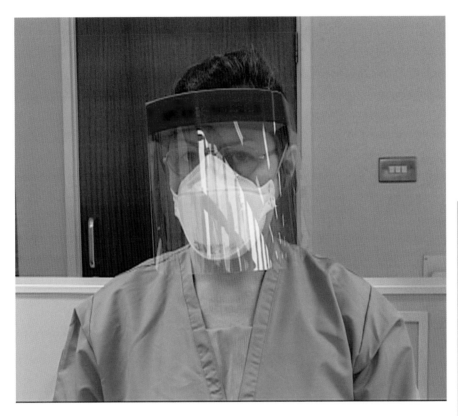

Figure 6.3 If the health care worker wears spectacles then a visor must be worn over the respirator mask. *Note*: A visor does not provide protection from respiratory aerosols, so a mask is worn under it.

- Visors are usually single-use disposable, but if designated reusable, then follow manufacturer's instructions for cleaning the surface with disinfectant

- Use disposable visors if treating patients with a contagious respiratory illness (e.g. flu), as reusable visors and goggles with elastic straps cannot be easily cleaned

The World Health Organization (WHO) recommends that PPE should be donned and removed in the following order to minimise self and environmental contamination:

Best practice guide: donning protective equipment

- Perform hand hygiene
- Put on fluid-resistant gown or plastic apron (if required)

- Put on surgical mask or (if appropriate) disposable particulate respirator
- Perform user seal check of particulate respirator
- Put on face shield or goggles
- Put on gloves (make sure that gloves cover cuff of disposable gown sleeves)

Removing protective equipment

- Remove gloves and discard in hazardous waste sack (gloves may be peeled from hands with a surgical gown as it is removed)
- Remove apron or gown
- Remove protective eyewear (goggles or face shield) and discard in hazardous waste container or decontaminate if reusable
- Remove mask or particulate respirator by grasping elastic bands or ties; do not touch front of mask or particulate respirator and discard in hazardous waste container (when working with a patient with pandemic flu then the mask/respirator is removed after the operator has left the treatment area)
- Perform hand hygiene

Gloves are removed first as they are contaminated on their outer surface with the patient's secretions and this manoeuvre then prevents you from touching and potentially infecting your own skin, eyes or mouth whilst removing the other contaminated items of PPE. Gloves should be removed immediately after completing treatment even if other items of PPE are not removed to prevent contamination of inanimate surfaces in the surgery environment.

TUNICS AND UNIFORMS

Prevent tunics and uniforms becoming a source of infection.

Uniform styles

After a day working in the surgery, tunics, trousers and uniforms will have become progressively contaminated with microbes from several sources including the wearer's skin organisms, the patient's pathogens and environmental microorganisms. In hospital wards, multi-drug-resistant bacteria (*Staphylococcus aureus*, *Clostridium difficile* and vancomycin-resistant enterococci) have been transmitted from patient to patient via contaminated uniforms, but transmission via this route appears to be rare (Wilson *et al.*, 2007).

In dentistry, splatter generated during the use of rotary equipment falls mainly on the operator's face, chest, hands and wrists. High-necked tunics and uniforms that cover the upper chest area are therefore advised. Neck ties have been implicated in transmission of MRSA and ties (except for bow ties) should not be worn when treating patients or if worn should be concealed under the tunic and uniform.

The current mantra is for working 'bare below the elbows', i.e. short sleeves, with no watches or jewellery in order to facilitate effective hand hygiene. Long sleeves become wet during hand washing and wet fabric promotes the survival and growth of bacteria. Dangling cuffs are also vulnerable to direct contamination by aerosols generated by the handpieces and respiratory droplets expelled from the patient's mouth. Remember however, when wearing short-sleeve uniforms, that the wrists and forearms will be covered with microbes after dental treatment and will need to be cleaned thoroughly.

Best practice guide: workwear code

- Protective clothing should not be worn in designated eating and rest areas within the practice. Remove protective clothing when eating and drinking

- Tunics and uniforms should be removed before leaving the practice and placed in an impermeable bag. Do not 'greet' friends and family with pathogens picked up in the surgery

- It is strongly recommended that tunics and uniforms are changed and washed daily

- When purchasing uniforms, it makes sense to choose fabrics and colours that can tolerate washing at the higher temperatures required to kill bacteria

- Wash uniforms using a 'hot' washing machine cycle at a setting of 60°C. This temperature will destroy most bacteria except heat-resistant spore formers

- Detergents release microbes and dirt from the fabric, which are then removed in the rinse water. Avoid overloading the machine as this will reduce the dilution effect of rinsing

- Iron the uniform, as the heat generated by ironing will help to destroy any bacteria remaining on the clothes. Ironing without prior washing reduces microbial counts by approximately 10^7 cfu/mL

- If dental staff wear their own clothes in the dental practice then similar hygiene measures should be employed

> *Tunic and uniforms are not ppe.*

Tunics and uniforms are not considered PPE as they are usually made of materials such as poly-cottons that are permeable to microorganisms and body fluids. Uniforms are not a substitute for PPE. Rather uniforms reflect the practice's corporate image and fulfil the patient's expectation of how a clinician should be dressed. If a risk assessment suggests that PPE is required to protect either the patient or the wearer then an impermeable gown or plastic apron should be worn over the uniform.

PROTECTIVE BARRIERS – PLASTIC APRONS AND SURGICAL GOWNS

Plastic aprons

> *Protect yourself from splatter with a disposable plastic apron.*

National and international recommendations on standard precautions recommend that health care workers wear disposable plastic aprons to protect the front of their uniform/clothing from microbial contamination arising from close contact with patients, materials and contaminated equipment or splatter. They are considered suitable for general clinical use, manually instrument cleaning or mopping up body fluid spills. If extensive exposure to blood is expected then disposable gowns are more appropriate.

Plastic aprons are classified as single-use items and should be changed between patients or each procedure and then discarded as hazardous clinical waste. They are prone to develop static electric charge in use, which attracts increased numbers of bacteria onto the apron. So, care must be taken to minimise touching the outer surface of the apron during wear or disposal; however, antistatic versions are available. Stocks of plastic aprons should be stored in a clean, dust-free place (Figure 6.4).

Surgical gowns

Conventional sterile surgical gowns or 'greens' have dual purpose. They are intended both to protect the patient from microorganisms shed from health care personnel during invasive surgery and to reduce the risk to the operator from contamination with blood and other body fluids. Commensal skin organisms

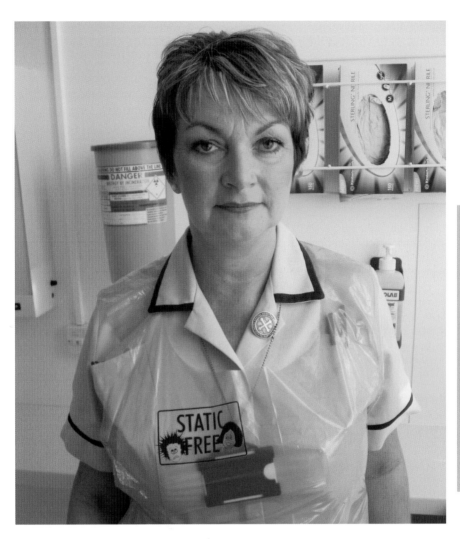

Figure 6.4 Antistatic disposable apron.

shed by the wearer account for approximately a third of the microorganism recovered from gowns. Higher counts are found below the waist. A working group established by the Hospital Infection Society concluded that theatre gowns and drapes should be made of waterproof disposable material. Disposables were more consistent in their performance as a barrier to microbes than reusable surgical linens. Purchase single-use gowns that comply with the European Standard EN 13795 as they resist tearing, wetting and bacterial penetration and dispersal.

In dentistry, disposable, full-length, impermeable, fluid-repellent surgical gowns are recommended where there is a high risk of blood splashes such as during minor oral surgery or implant surgery. Gowns are usually the first piece of PPE to be donned after hand hygiene has been performed. Gowns should have long sleeves with tight-fitting cuffs. Gloves are worn over the cuff of the sleeve, which protects the wrists from contamination and helps to prevent wetting of the cuff. When removing the gown, the outer, 'contaminated', side of the gown is turned inwards and rolled into a bundle, and then discarded into hazardous waste receptacle.

REFERENCES AND WEBSITES

Lipp, A. and Edwards, P. (2002). Disposable surgical face masks for preventing surgical wound infection in clean surgery. *Cochrane Database of Systematic Reviews*, Issue 1. Art. No.: CD002929. DOI: 10.1002/14651858.CD002929.

Seto, W.H., Tsang, D., Yung, R.W.H. *et al.* (2003). Effectiveness of precautions against droplets and contact in prevention of nosocomial transmission of severe acute respiratory syndrome (SARS). *Lancet*, 361, 1519–1520.

Wilson, J.A., Loveday, H.P., Hoffman, P.N. and Pratt, R.J. (2007). Uniform: an evidence review of the microbiological significance of uniforms and uniform policy in the prevention and control of healthcare-associated infections. Report to the Department of Health (England). *Journal of Hospital Infection*, 66, 301–307.

Further reading

National Institute for Health and Clinical Excellence (NICE) (June 2003). *Clinical Guideline 2 Infection control Prevention of Healthcare-Associated Infection in Primary and Community Care*. Available at http://www.nice.org.uk.

Pratt, R.J., Pellowea, C.M., Wilson, J.A. *et al.* (2007). Epic2: National evidence-based guidelines for preventing healthcare-associated infections in NHS Hospitals in England. *Journal of Hospital Infection*, 65S, S1–S64.

Chapter 7

Sterilization and disinfection of dental instruments

DECONTAMINATION CYCLE

Decontamination is carried out for two important reasons:

- To make a reusable device safe for staff to handle

- To minimise (disinfection) or eliminate (sterilization) the risk of cross-infection from person to person by direct contact

The ultimate goal is to produce a sterile instrument that is completely free of all microorganisms. Sterilization is not sufficient on its own to achieve this aim. Instruments cannot be sterilised unless they are first cleaned because debris (cement, blood, lubricant oil etc.) adhering to the surface of an instrument can inhibit or interfere with the sterilization process. Therefore, decontamination is an incremental process with each stage (see Figure 7.1) contributing to the killing and removal of microorganisms.

Definitions:

- *Cleaning*: physical removal (including prions) but not necessarily killing of microbes

- *Disinfection*: reduction of the microbial load to a level that makes the disinfected object safe to handle

- *Sterilization*: killing and removal of all microorganisms including bacterial spores

Vegetative (non-spore-forming) bacteria, fungi, viruses and protozoa are readily killed at temperatures above 60–65°C. Spore-forming bacteria and *Mycobacteria* spp. have protective cell walls that make them relatively resistant to thermal killing. To destroy the organisms, the higher temperatures generated during sterilization are necessary, whereas prions are highly resistant to thermal killing and are mainly removed during cleaning and disinfection. Complete removal of bacteria is an essential component of the process, as endotoxin a breakdown product derived from the cell wall of dead Gram-negative bacteria,

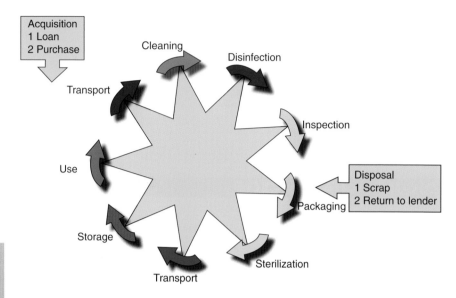

Figure 7.1 Decontamination cycle of reusable instruments (courtesy of Paul Morris).

though not infectious, can trigger an inflammatory reaction that ranges from mild to sometimes fatal toxic shock. In addition to removal of endotoxin, a decontaminated instrument whether it has been disinfected or sterilised should be free from:

- Residues of previous clinical treatment, e.g. cement, microbes, blood and human tissue

- Residues from the decontamination process, e.g. disinfectants and limescale

- Contamination by dust, dirt and environmental microbial contamination

WHY HAS CLEANING BECOME SO IMPORTANT?

Prion proteins are more resistant to sterilization.

Cleaning has always been an important component of the decontamination process, but has increased in significance as a result of the prion disease vCJD (variant Creutzfeldt–Jakob disease) appearing in the humans in the mid-1990s (see Chapter 2). Prion diseases are rare, infectious, fatal, neurodegenerative disorders, which present as sporadic, familial or acquired disease. The infectious agents are prions. Unlike other pathogens, they contain no genetic material

STERILIZATION AND DISINFECTION OF DENTAL INSTRUMENTS

in the form of DNA or RNA, but instead are composed of a protein with an abnormal conformation. Proteins are considerably more resistant to the thermal denaturation than DNA or RNA. Sterilization reduces infectivity (i.e. deactivation of prion agents) only by a 100- to 1000-fold. There is evidence to suggest that prions are modified by adsorption onto a metal surface making them more resistant to decontamination. In most infections, the organism has to be released from the surface of a surgical instrument into the patient's bloodstream or tissues to initiate an infection. This sequence of events is unnecessary for transmission of prion disease, as infection can occur even when prion agent remains adherent to the instrument. Once present on an instrument, the prion can continue to infect patients until it is physically removed.

At present, there are no modifications to the sterilization processes available for routine use, which can inactivate prion protein without having a detrimental impact on instrument integrity. Radiofrequency-generated gas plasma and enzymic disinfectants, which are undergoing experimental evaluation, look promising and may in the future be employed to deactivate prions. Currently, cleaning which physically removes protein has become of prime importance in the decontamination cycle. Previously, the benchmark standard for cleaning was 'the reduction of bacterial load', and now it has been raised to the 'removal of prion proteins'. On a practical level, this change is translated into the replacement of manual cleaning by automated cleaning, preferably with a thermal washer disinfector. However dedicated the person cleaning the dental instruments, all manual procedures are subject to operator variation as a result of time constraints or tiredness. Automated cleaning has the major advantage of being reproducible and open to validation.

LEGAL REQUIREMENTS AND TECHNICAL STANDARDS FOR DECONTAMINATION

Complying with the law

Sterilisers and thermal washer disinfectors are classed under the law as medical devices. Both the equipment and the site where decontamination takes place are required to operate according to EEC Medical Devices Directive (MDD) 93/42/EEC. In the UK, the directive is translated into the Medical Devices Regulations (MDR) 2002 under the Consumer Protection Act. The regulations apply specifically to large sterile services departments supplying hospitals with sterile reusable instruments. But under the Health Act 2006 (Hygiene Code – see Chapter 1), the basic principles affecting control of the decontamination process and the working environment apply to all health care facilities including dental practices (see Table 7.1).

STERILIZATION AND DISINFECTION OF DENTAL INSTRUMENTS

Table 7.1 Hygiene code

Summary of regulations affecting reusable instrument decontamination:

- Proper account is taken of the relevant national guidelines

- Decontamination of reusable medical devices takes place in appropriate dedicated facilities

- Appropriate procedures are used for the acquisition and maintenance of decontamination equipment

- Staff are trained in decontamination processes and hold appropriate competencies for their role

- There is a monitoring system in place to ensure that decontamination processes are fit for purpose and meet the required standard

Technical standards for decontamination

European technical standards for sterilisers and washer disinfectors were recently revised and upgraded. In the UK, to reflect theses changes and to bring them into line with the new British/European standards, BS EN ISO 15883 (washer disinfectors) and BS EN ISO 13060 (benchtop sterilisers), all the technical and operating guidance was united into a single document called Decontamination Series HTM 01. Part 05 of the series 'Decontamination in Dentistry' governs activities in general dental practice (available from www.decontamination.nhs.uk), which is monitored by the Healthcare Commission, UK. They take the Hygiene Code as their benchmark for audit purposes (see Table 7.1). As dental practices like other health care organisations are required to take into account all relevant national guidelines, dental practice staff are obliged to be familiar with the content of these documents. In addition, they should follow the guidance on setting up a decontamination room and operating equipment such as sterilisers.

WHERE SHOULD INSTRUMENT DECONTAMINATION TAKE PLACE?

Currently, sterilization of equipment for use in dentistry takes place within the dental practice, but this is not the only option available.

Options:

1. Outsource decontamination to an accredited sterile services department

2. Use CE-marked single-use medical devices

Table 7.2 Key points for organising decontamination in the dental practice

- Ensure that there is an effective management control system decontamination
- Nominate a lead person with responsibility for decontamination in the practice with line management responsibility to the practice owner
- Have documented decontamination policies
- Procure equipment compatible with decontamination load
- Undertake sterilization in dedicated facilities outside the patient treatment room
- Restrict manual cleaning to those items incompatible with automated processes. Clean compatible instruments using an automated process, e.g. thermal washer disinfector and ultrasonic bath
- Decontamination equipment must be fit for purpose. Fully validate equipment before use. Perform maintenance, service and periodic testing in accordance with current recommendations
- Track and trace instrument sets through decontamination processes and to the patient
- Retain all documentation in preparation for external audit or inspections
- Operate a documented training scheme and keep individual training records for all personnel involved in decontamination

Compiled from HTM 01-01 and HTM 01-05.

3. Undertake local decontamination to national standards (HTM 01-01 and HTM 01-05)

4. Combination of 1–3

Most, but not all, dental practices will probably opt for option 4, i.e. to continue local decontamination combined with selective use of disposable instruments. As we have seen in the previous section, this puts the onus on the dental practice to comply with the national standards which are outlined in brief in Table 7.2. Note that validation of the decontamination cycle is considered as important as the design of the decontamination room and the type of equipment used within it. The next part of this chapter will outline how this can be achieved.

DESIGN OF DEDICATED DECONTAMINATION UNITS

Ideally, the treatment room should be used exclusively for clinical treatment and should not be used for any part of the decontamination cycle including storage of instruments. Why is this? Primarily, to ensure both patient safety and quality assurance of the sterilization process. To ensure that each step of the decontamination process reduces the load of microbes on the instruments, it is crucial

STERILIZATION AND DISINFECTION OF DENTAL INSTRUMENTS

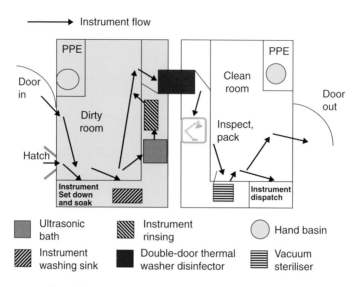

Figure 7.2 Basic design for a two-room decontamination facility.

that clean and dirty instruments are segregated and are not recontaminated after cleaning or sterilization by direct contact, splashes and aerosols. Moving sterilization out of the treatment area protects the patient from contaminated aerosols generated during cleaning instruments used on previous patients. A steriliser is a pressurised item of equipment and the pressure that builds up behind the door of the steriliser is equivalent to 750 kg or three-quarters of a tonne. If the door fails, which occasionally happens, then the steriliser effectively becomes a bomb, doing considerable damage to anything in its path. If the steriliser is housed on the work surface in a small surgery, the patient or members of the dental team could be seriously hurt.

All theses requirements can be met with a dedicated decontamination facility. Segregation between those instruments awaiting decontamination and disinfected and sterile instruments can be achieved in several ways:

- A two-room decontamination facility with one room for dirty instruments and the other room for cleaned instruments for sterilization. A double-door washer disinfector is placed in the barrier between the dirty and clean rooms (see Figure 7.2). The design includes controlled access to the rooms for authorised trained staff with a hand-through hatch (for the delivery of dirty sets of instruments and equipment). This is the preferred option as cross-contamination is very unlikely to occur. The design most closely mimics the tried-and-tested layout used in hospital sterile services departments.

- A single-room decontamination facility (see Figure 7.3) with a one-way flow of instruments and pattern of working from dirty to clean. Thermal washer

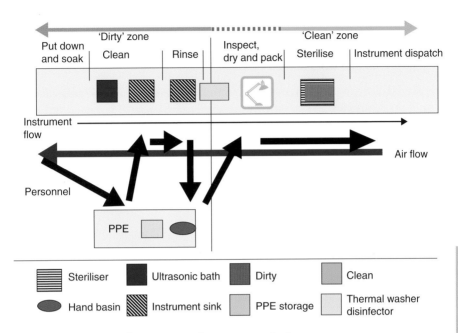

Figure 7.3 Basic design for a one-room decontamination facility.

disinfector is placed in between dirty and clean areas. To prevent aerosol cross-contamination, the room will need to be ventilated by a controlled airflow in the direction opposite to that of the instruments, i.e. from clean to dirty. This is not foolproof as airflows can be disrupted by opening the doors or windows, so this is not the preferred option. Figure 7.3 shows movement patterns of staff within the room to maintain the zoning. This requires a high level of staff discipline and training to achieve this work flow and therefore more prone to human error than a two-room facility.

In both options, instruments are transported to and from the treatment room in a clean box with a secure lid. Staff are advised to clean hands and put on personal protective equipment (PPE) on entering the decontamination facility and remove PPE and clean hands on exiting. They are advised to change gloves and aprons when shifting from working in the dirty to the clean zone to prevent cross-contamination of the two processes. Decontamination rooms should contain the following features.

Basic requirements

- Controlled access doors
- Preferably an instrument pass-through hatch

- Uncluttered, single run of sealed, easily cleaned worktop which makes working and surface disinfection easier

- Hand basin and storage for PPE (see Chapter 6)

- Filtered clean air flow to prevent contamination (this includes both microbes and dust particles)

Dirty room/zone (instrument cleaning)

- A setting down area for dirty instruments and precleaning soaking of instruments

- Ultrasonic bath

- A deep instrument-washing sink with detergent dispenser

- A rinsing sink

- Thermal washer disinfector

Clean room/zone (inspection, sterilization and storage)

- A setting down area for machine-washed instruments, with suitable lighting for instrument inspection (e.g. checking for visible contamination and instrument functionality/damage)

- Instrument wrapping (if using a vacuum steriliser)

- A steam steriliser (vacuum and/or non-vacuum)

- An area for setting down (and wrapping if instruments sterilised in non-vacuum steriliser)

- Controlled access to the clean room as repeated door opening hinders environmental control

Sterile instrument storage

Storage of instruments must be away from the patient treatment area and it has been recommended that they should also be stored outside of the decontamination room (Scottish Health Planning Note 13, Part 2, Decontamination Facilities: Local Decontamination Units, NHS National Services Scotland, June 2008; www.hfs.scot.nhs/uk/publications).

- Cleanable shelving or racking (covered) for storing sterilised instruments in procedure-based trays, wrapped cassettes or pouches, with orderly storage to facilitate stock control

- Separate sterile wrapped instruments from instruments that are packaged post-sterilization, which are non-sterile and have a shorter storage life

The actual design will vary with the space available in the dental practice.

Temporal separation

The illustrated designs are for 'ideal' decontamination facilities and the interpretation of the Medical Devices Directive is not uniform across the European Union. But the same best practice principles of segregation of dirty and clean procedures apply even when the decontamination is performed in the treatment room, as patient safety is paramount. In the latter situation, a degree of separation can be achieved by introducing some simple measures. Temporal separation (separating activities in time) can be used to conduct different activities in the same space. Patient safety can be enhanced by not decontaminating instrument whilst the patient is in the treatment room. Most surgeries have two sinks: one for the nurse and the other for the dentist, and one of these can be designated as the dedicated sink for instrument cleaning. Recontamination of instruments can be reduced by thorough surface disinfection or worktops between dirty and clean stages. Adequate ventilation and exhaust air extraction with 8–10 air changes per hour in the treatment room will help to reduce air contamination to a low level.

However, such an approach would not be considered acceptable in the UK except as an interim measure before a planned move into a dedicated decontamination facility. The size of the dental practice is not considered as an excuse for omission of any of the fundamental principles of segregation and separation of clean and dirty instruments. Practices which have limited space may consider outsourcing their instrument decontamination to a sterile services provider.

Purchasing of dental equipment

Dental devices marketed in the European Union carry a 'CE' mark, which indicates that the equipment is 'fit for the intended purpose'. Manufacturers of medical/dental devices must by law provide decontamination instructions including methods for cleaning, disinfection, sterilization and state any limit to the number of times an item can be sterilised. Before purchasing a new item, it is prudent to check the manufacturer's decontamination instructions to ensure that the instruments can be decontaminated with the facilities, that you have, available in the practice. Give preference when choosing instruments to those that can be cleaned by using automated methods, e.g. thermal washer disinfector (see Figure 7.4); alternatively, consider a single-use instrument for difficult-to-clean instruments.

STERILIZATION AND DISINFECTION
OF DENTAL INSTRUMENTS

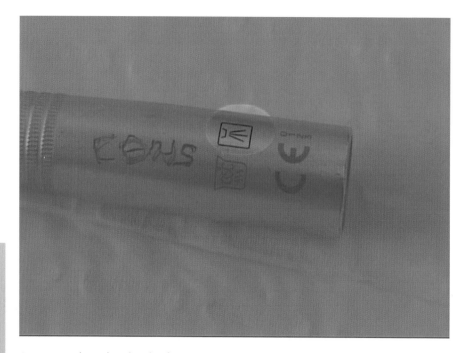

Figure 7.4 Thermal washer disinfector safe symbol on a dental handpiece.

PRESTERILIZATION CLEANING OF DENTAL INSTRUMENTS

The effectiveness of the sterilization process depends upon direct contact between the steam and all surfaces of the load. Residual human tissues, oil or other deposits will prevent contact between the steam and the surfaces of the load. Unremoved contaminants can become fixed to the instruments during sterilization making subsequent removal more difficult. Therefore, all items that you intend to sterilise must be clean and dry before you place them in the steriliser chamber.

Automated versus manual cleaning

Instruments can be cleaned manually or by machine using an ultrasonic bath and/or a thermal washer disinfector. Manual cleaning of instruments should be restricted to those items incompatible with automated washing. Studies have demonstrated that washer disinfectors are more efficient at reducing the bacterial load during pre-sterilization cleaning than either ultrasonic cleaning or manual cleaning of dental instruments. Staff safety is enhanced as instruments do not need to be scrubbed, so there is less exposure to pathogenic microorganisms, sharps injuries or noxious chemicals. Overall productivity is increased in the dental practice as more time becomes available for clinical activities. There are some disadvantages to thermal disinfectors. Manual cleaning is faster than using a thermal washer disinfector. Downtime for instruments cleaned and dried in a thermal washer disinfector and sterilised in a vacuum steriliser is approximately 2 hours, necessitating the purchase of additional instruments if the same number of patients are to be seen.

Preventing corrosion of instruments

Proteins in blood and saliva left on the instrument after treatment are absorbed and then fixed onto the surface of the instrument. Fixation is a chemical process that takes about 40 minutes at room temperature, but is faster at higher temperatures. Eventually, blood and saline will corrode stainless steel instruments, leading to pitting and rusting of the surface. Damaged and pitted instruments are more difficult to clean effectively and corrosion may reduce the life of the instrument. Ideally, instruments should be cleaned as soon as possible after use. If it is not practical to clean the instruments immediately then soak them in a non-ionic or enzymatic detergent solution, or precleaning foam.

Manual cleaning of instruments

> *Manual cleaning carries a sharps injury and inhalation risk.*

Use a non-foaming, neutral (pH 5–9) detergent dispensed in a measured dose in a measured volume of water for manual cleaning or ultrasonic baths. Always take great care with sharp instruments. Before cleaning the instruments the member of staff should put on the following protective clothing:

- Disposable apron/gown
- Face shield or face mask
- Household gloves (surgical gloves should not be worn)
- When moving from working in a designated dirty area to a clean area, change gloves and plastic apron and clean hands

Best practice guide: manual instruments cleaning

- Dedicated deep sinks (separate washing and rinsing sinks) located in a designated dirty zone

- Use a non-foaming detergent (do *not* use washing-up liquid, which leaves a residue and the surface foam impedes visibility of sharp instruments)

- Use nylon brushes, not green pads or wire brushes. Cleaning equipment (e.g. brushes) should be cleaned and sterilised (or alternatively use disposables) and stored dry between use. Brushes should not be stored in disinfectant solutions

- Use non-shedding and disposable cloths for cleaning and drying equipment

- Fill basin with lukewarm water (water hotter than 35°C will coagulate proteins and inhibit their removal)

- Fully immerse instruments and clean below the waterline to reduce aerosol formation. Avoid scrubbing under running water

- Disassemble multi-part instruments; pay attention to crevices and joints

- Final rinse under hot water to aid instrument drying

- Dry instruments to prevent carryover of contaminated wash water into the steriliser

- Visually inspect instruments for residual debris or blood after cleaning and repeat if necessary

CLEANING OF DENTAL HANDPIECES

Automated dental handpiece cleaning

Dental handpiece can be cleaned manually or preferably by automated cleaning either using a pre-sterilization dental handpiece cleaning machine or using a thermal washer disinfector. Many of the contralateral, straight and turbine handpieces currently available are thermal washer disinfectors which are safe and carry the washer disinfector symbol (see Figure 7.4). Thermal washer disinfectors are fitted with plug-in connectors for dental handpieces that ensure that the internal lumens are disinfected. If recommended by the manufacturer, lubricate the bearings with service oil after the thermal washer disinfector stage.

A dental handpiece cleaning typical machine cleans the air and water channels with the aid of a detergent spray solution, followed by cleaning and lubricating the bearings and gears with oil. Finally, the excess oil is purged, which reduces the amount of carryover of oil into the steriliser, the interior is dried with compressed air and the handpiece is ready for sterilization.

If opting to clean the handpiece manually, then avoid immersing it in an ultrasonic bath or a chlorine-containing disinfectant as this will cause corrosion. Instead, wipe carefully the outer surface of the handpiece using an alcohol wipe leaving sufficient time for evaporation. Dry the water channel with compressed air and outer casing with a non-linting cloth and then spray service oil once (approximately 1 second) through the lumen onto a disposable soft paper towel. Place handpiece with the head downwards in a rack to drain off excess oil.

MECHANICAL CLEANING WITH AN ULTRASONIC BATH

Ultrasonic baths are significantly more effective than manual cleaning.

Ultrasonic cleaning works by cavitation generated by high-frequency sound waves that create regions of alternating high and low pressure in the bath. Bubbles form in the detergent under low-pressure implode when the pressure changes from low to high, dislodging debris from nooks and crannies and cleaning the surface. Water absorbs oxygen and this is released as bubbles of oxygen gas, which interfere with the cleaning action of the bath. To avoid this problem, degas the detergent solution by running the bath empty for a few minutes before immersing the instruments.

Ultrasonic baths are an effective method for cleaning intricate, jointed or serrated stainless steel and metal instruments and items that are heavily soiled, e.g. with cement. Plastic instruments are not successfully cleaned by this method as they absorb the ultrasonic energy. Remember that the ultrasonic baths only clean and remove microorganisms; they do not disinfect instruments as the running temperature is below the minimum required to kill even vegetative bacteria.

Best practice guide: using an ultrasonic bath

- Rinse off blood or other cross-contamination by immersing instruments under warm water

- Place instruments in a basket. Open or dismantle instruments, if appropriate

- Use manufacturer's default temperature setting or, if bath requires, manual temperature setting (typical programme is 20–40°C for 3 minutes, which minimises the rate of coagulation of proteinaceous material)

- Use a low-foaming enzymic detergent effective at low temperatures at the manufacturer's recommended concentration and dose

- Rinse thoroughly to remove detergent residues by immersing in clean water (unless machine has an automatic rinse cycle) and dry

- Inspect instruments for residual debris after cleaning and repeat, if necessary

STERILIZATION AND DISINFECTION OF DENTAL INSTRUMENTS

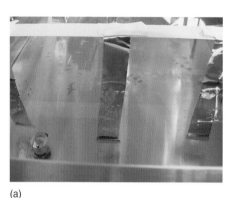
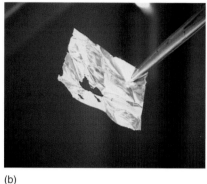

(a)   (b)

Figure 7.5 (a) Foil strip suspended across an ultrasonic bath. (b) Closeup demonstrating pitting and perforation of the foil indicating that the ultrasonic bath is working satisfactorily. (Photographs supplied by Paul Jenkins.)

Best practice guide: maintenance and validation of ultrasonic bath

- Ultrasonic bath solution becomes contaminated with debris, so empty bath every 4 hours or before if the solution becomes visibly heavily contaminated

- Only operate with the lid onto avoid aerosol contamination

- Empty, clean and dry bath at the end of the session/day

- Perform a quarterly *validation test* to confirm ultrasonic action, e.g. the aluminium foil test. A series of 5 cm^2 foil strip is suspended in the bath for 3 minutes (see Figure 7.5(a)). Inspect the foil. The edges of the foil should be serrated with pitting and/or perforation of centre of the strip (see Figure 7.5(b)). Record the test results in the machine logbook

- Get the bath regularly serviced and tested by a suitably qualified engineer (see HTM 01-05)

THERMAL WASHER DISINFECTORS

> *Washer disinfectors provide automated, reproducible and validated cleaning.*

Most thermal washer disinfectors have an operating cycle that includes a cool prewash (below 35°C to prevent protein coagulation and remove debris), main wash, rinse, thermal disinfection and post-disinfection rinse. Thermal disinfection is achieved by the use of hot water (set at 90°C for 1 minute; EN ISO standard 15883) coming into direct contact with the instruments and equipment

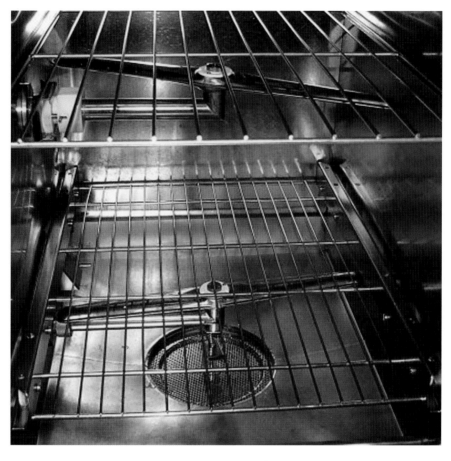

Figure 7.6 Scaling and staining of the interior walls and floor of a thermal washer disinfector which has been connected to an unsuitable water supply; compare the sheen on the horizontal shelf to the staining of the other surfaces. (Photograph supplied by Paul Jenkins.)

STERILIZATION AND DISINFECTION
OF DENTAL INSTRUMENTS

for a specified period of time, followed by a drying cycle. Thermal disinfection reduces the number of viable microorganisms contaminating the devices, but may not necessarily inactivate some viruses and bacterial spores, so instruments are not sterile at the end of the programme. A high-quality water such as reverse osmosis (RO) water is recommended for the final rinse as this reduces level of total dissolved solids left on the instruments as a residue. Mains water used for the final rinse will recontaminate the load and promote biofilm formation inside the machine. RO water though not strictly sterile is virtually free of pathogens and endotoxins. In hard-water areas, the water should be softened (Figure 7.6). Machines are designed with independent 'watchdog circuits' that monitor the detergent dosing verification, detergent cleaning cycle and thermal disinfection cycle. They are programmed to alert the operator of any failures or malfunctions, and will abort the cycle if errors are detected. An integrated printer provides a permanent record of the operation parameters and performance indicators of the disinfection cycle. Domestic dishwashers are not an acceptable alternative. They do not perform to the same specifications as the washer disinfectors do; they may not adequately clean the inner surface of hollow or lumened instruments, and nor are they capable of validation in accordance with HTM 01-01 and HTM 01-05 (see www.decontamination.gov.uk for additional guidance on validation testing and protocols).

Trays/cassettes are available that are suitable for use in a thermal washer disinfector, steriliser and for storage. Using such systems significantly reduces the amount of instrument handling and will reduce the incident of sharps injuries and aid traceability.

INSTRUMENT INSPECTION

Instruments should be function tested as part of the decontamination process. Instruments that are damaged should be repaired or taken out of service. Instruments that develop or sustain surface damage due to general wear, pitting or corrosion encourage dirt and bacteria to accumulate and are more difficult to clean and sterilise effectively. Furthermore, they may be more prone to failing during function and could potentially harm patients or staff.

DENTAL INSTRUMENT STERILIZATION

Sterilization is the stage in the decontamination, targeting the killing and removal of microbial contamination, in particular bacterial spores. Invasive instruments need to be sterile at the time of use to prevent infection of the oral tissues and the transfer of microorganisms from person to person. Therefore, benchtop steam steriliser used in the dental practice must be suitable for the intended loads, and be validated before use, maintained and operated properly to ensure that the load is sterilised on every occasion.

SUITABILITY OF STERILISER FOR DIFFERENT LOADS

Never sterilise heat-sensitive items or single-use items in any type of steriliser.

There are three main types of benchtop sterilisers available for use in dentistry, namely the N-type non-vacuum (also known as downward displacement/ gravity displacement) sterilisers and the B- and S-type vacuum benchtop

Table 7.3 Suitability of sterilisers for different types of instruments

Type	Air removal	Suitability for different types of instruments
N	**Passive** (gravity displacement)	Solid, non-wrapped
B	**Active air removal** by vacuum pulse	All types of equipment including hollow (e.g. forceps), lumened (e.g. dental handpieces), wrapped and porous (e.g. swabs)
S	**Active air removal** by vacuum super-atmospheric pulsing; steam injection through lumen	Only suitable for loads specified by manufacturer

sterilisers. The suitability of these three types of sterilisers for different types of equipment is summarised in Table 7.3. Steam sterilization relies on complete air removal in order for the steam to come into intimate contact with the entire surface of a device within the chamber. Non-vacuum phase sterilisers rely on passive displacement of the air by the steam, which when used for instruments with lumens may result in inadequate air removal from the interior of the instrument and a failure to sterilise. Unfortunately, cases of serious infection have ensued when such incompletely sterilised instruments were used on vulnerable patients. Hence, N-type sterilisers are intended for the processing of solid, non-wrapped equipment for immediate use. B-type sterilisers are suitable for hollow and solid instruments as the air is removed actively with the aid of a vacuum phase. A post-sterilization drying stage ensures that the load is dry before the door is opened, allowing the instruments to be wrapped or pouched. However, this prolongs the total cycle time considerably.

STERILISER INSTALLATION AND VALIDATION

A new steriliser has to be installed, commissioned and validated before you use it by an accredited engineer and the results retained (for a minimum of 2 years) in the steriliser logbook for future reference. All steam sterilisers and associated pipework are subject to the Pressure Systems Safety Regulations 2000 as these can be dangerous items of equipment unless regularly maintained and examined by a suitably accredited engineer (see Chapter 1). An engineer (also referred to as a 'competent person' in the technical literature) will draw up a written examination schedule that is based on the age of the equipment. Under the regulations, staff are to be fully trained in the operation and use of the equipment and the management of steam-related injuries (scalds/burns) and instructions for emergencies. You must have pressure vessel liability insurance for both your steriliser(s) and compressor(s) to cover against accidents caused by pressurised equipment and steam.

STERILIZATION AND DISINFECTION OF DENTAL INSTRUMENTS

Table 7.4 Sterilization temperature bands, holding times and pressures for steam sterilization

Sterilization temperature range: minimum (°C)	Sterilization temperature range: maximum (°C)	Approximate pressure (bar)	Minimum hold time (minutes)
134	137	2.25	3
126	129	1.50	10
121	124	1.15	15

SELECTING THE CORRECT TEMPERATURE, PRESSURE AND TIME FOR STERILIZATION

When selecting the temperature for sterilization, use the highest temperature compatible with the load, normally 134–137°C for a holding time of 3 minutes at a pressure of 2.5 bar (normally the default setting on sterilisers). Alternative time, pressure and temperatures suitable for sterilization are shown in Table 7.4.

STEAM PURITY AND MAINTENANCE OF WATER RESERVOIR CHAMBER

All sterilisers have a reservoir chamber from which the water is delivered for steam generation. Tap water is not recommended as it contains dissolved minerals which can cause scaling of the heating element and the chamber, adversely effecting the normal functioning of the steriliser. The water needs to be of high quality to safeguard both the patient and the steriliser. Reservoir water and steam should be free of pathogens and endotoxins (pyrogen) with low, specified amounts of inorganic minerals. Bacteria in the reservoir water are killed during the steam generation process, but the endotoxins (lipopolysaccharide) released from the bacterial cell walls remain, and as the water in the steam condenses on cooling, it coats the instruments with endotoxins. Bacterial endotoxins are biologically active even when the bacteria from which they are released are dead. Endotoxins cause hypersensitivity reactions, toxic shock and periodontal disease and can inhibit wound healing.

Types of water and steam purity

Suitable types of water that have the desired properties include *sterile water for irrigation BP* and certain RO waters of equivalent specification. RO water is made by forcing water through a series of semipermeable membranes under pressure to remove minerals and endotoxins. Bacteria are removed with bacterial filters or ultraviolet light treatment. RO water can be purchased commercially or made on site in the dental surgery. Small on-site RO machines can be plumbed directly into the steriliser and the washer disinfector. RO machines need to be maintained and the water periodically sampled and tested for chemical contaminants, mineral content and pH.

Purified waters such as *deionised* or *distilled* waters can also be made in the dental practice. The disadvantage of the latter two types of water is that although they have low levels of mineral content the actual amount is unknown. They are commonly contaminated with endotoxins and pathogens, but at unspecified levels, so their quality cannot be guaranteed.

Partially used bottles of water or locally produced waters should be discarded at the end of the day as the microbiological quality of all types of water deteriorates rapidly on storage. Bacteria divide approximately every 20 minutes and grow exponentially. So, starting with one bacterium in a bottle of water after a 7-hour working day there will be over 4 million bacteria – a veritable bacterial soup!

MAINTENANCE OF THE STERILISER WATER RESERVOIR

Problems associated with recycled water

Depending on the model of steriliser, water in the reservoir is either recycled or used once and discharged into the drain at the end of the sterilization cycle. If instruments are ineffectively cleaned and dried prior to sterilization, the recycled water will become progressively more contaminated by the end of each cycle with endotoxin and lubricant oil that is deposited on subsequent loads. Single-use water cycle sterilisers are a preferable option as they avoid this problem.

Biofilm formation in the water reservoir

As the water cools in the reservoir, the temperatures become suitable for bacterial growth and a bacterial biofilm will form on the walls and floor of the chamber, contributing further to the accumulation of endotoxins (see Chapter 9 for an explanation of bacterial biofilm formation). Sampling of steriliser reservoirs in dental practices revealed that the bacterial count is in the order of 10^4–10^5 cfu/mL. After daily cleaning and refilling with fresh water the bacterial count and endotoxin titres were virtually eliminated. Evidence for the harmful effects of endotoxin comes from several reported outbreaks of postsurgical keratitis (a serious inflammatory condition resulting in some patients in loss of visual acuity). Endotoxin contamination was traced back to biofilms coating

STERILIZATION AND DISINFECTION OF DENTAL INSTRUMENTS

the steriliser reservoirs. The outbreaks ceased after the biofilm was removed. This was achieved by daily draining down of the reservoir, then cleaning and scrubbing of the reservoir chamber and finally rinsing with sterile water.

Best practice guide: daily maintenance of steriliser reservoir

- Fill with fresh (commercially or on-site produced) RO water

- Regularly disinfect the RO machine and validate the water quality according to the manufacturer's instructions

- Allow water to cool and then drain down and replenish water in the reservoir every 4 hours. Do not top up. Alternatively, use steriliser with single-use water cycle

- Dispose of partially used bottles or locally produced water at the end of the day (avoid storage of water)

- At the end of the day, wipe down the reservoir with sterile water (or 70% alcohol if recommended by the manufacturer), using a disposable lint-free cloth, dried and covered with a lid. Do not use a disinfectant as this can damage the pipework, unless specifically recommended by the manufacturer.

- Leave reservoir empty until future use

HOW DO YOU KNOW YOUR STERILISER IS WORKING?

Validation and periodic testing of the steriliser

Successful sterilization depends on consistent reproducibility of the sterilising conditions during every cycle. Sterilization is a process whose effectiveness cannot be guaranteed by inspection of the product. Process monitoring of individual sterilization cycles is the approved method for guaranteeing that instruments and equipment are sterile. This relies on the assumption that if all the contributory processes are correct (e.g. temperature, pressure and holding time) and well controlled then the desired outcome (sterile instruments) will result. This is referred to as the automatic control test (ACT), which is performed daily. The test results provide evidence that the steriliser is achieving sterilising conditions. A printout or a handwritten copy of the results should be kept as a permanent record in the logbook, providing a history of activity for the steriliser.

Microbiological spore testing to verify sterilization is used in some countries, but is not recommended in the UK as this method cannot provide immediate results on steriliser functioning and is prone to give false-positive results. Each steriliser in the practice should have its own logbook to record details of the installation, commissioning and validation, and maintenance history, including descriptions of breakdowns and time out of action. All records should be kept for a minimum of 2 years (HTM 01-05).

Daily automatic control test

The ACT requires the temperature and pressure profiles and the holding time of the cycle to be compared with the values obtained when the steriliser (vacuum or non-vacuum) was known to be working correctly (i.e. the specific settings for your steriliser which were calibrated by the engineer at the most recent validation. These settings will vary slightly for each steriliser). Perform the ACT using the sterilising cycle with the highest temperature compatible with the load (usually 134–137°C). The test is performed either with an empty chamber or with the load composition that is the same each day. A (paper or electronic) printer fitted to the sterilisers will record the results of the test for you, providing an accurate, permanent record and saving your time. If your steriliser does not have a printer fitted, observe the gauges and record the following during the sterilising (holding) stage of the cycle:

- Maximum values of the chamber temperatures and pressures indicated on the gauges

- Holding stage duration in minutes and seconds

The most important part of the test is to record in the logbook whether the steriliser passed or failed the test and should be signed and dated by the operator.

Test failures

The daily ACT results should be viewed as a medicolegal document; it is the only evidence you have that the steriliser was working and could protect you from litigation. A failure of the ACT indicates that the steriliser is not working correctly. The practice should have a written procedure for dealing with test failures and the steriliser should be withdrawn from service until the problem is rectified and a successful test achieved. In addition to the daily ACTs, keep the printer read out for every sterilization cycle to provide assurance that sterilised loads are being consistently produced.

Steam penetration test

A vacuum steriliser, because it has an active vacuum phase, requires additional daily testing in the form of the steam penetration test. This test checks that the air removal stage is effective and that any residual air and other

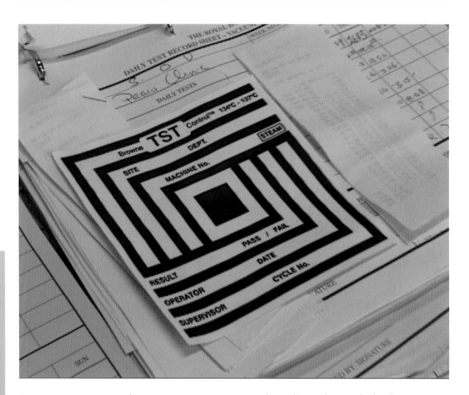

Figure 7.7 A Bowie–Dick steam penetration test inserted into the sterilization logbook.

non-condensable gases (NCGs) will not interfere with the sterilization process. It is essential to perform this test with only the steam penetration test device in the chamber. Anything else in the chamber will disrupt the test and produce an erroneous result. Only use the test pack specified by the manufacturer, e.g. Bowie and Dick type or manufacturer's equivalent steam penetration test kit (Helix test). Results (pass or fail and the test card) are recorded in the steriliser logbook and the data kept for a minimum of 2 years (Figure 7.7).

Chemical process indicators

Chemical process indicators include autoclave tape, test tubes, sterilization packaging or bags containing a chemical indicator. Typically, heat-sensitive chemical indicators react when exposed to steam and demonstrates a change in colour. Process indicators are designed to help you distinguish whether an instrument has been through a steriliser cycle (Figure 7.8). They offer *no* guarantee that the instrument is sterile. They should never be considered as an alternative to the ACT or cycle record. Process indicators will change colour if

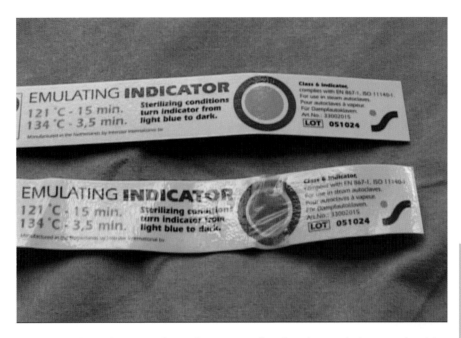

Figure 7.8 Chemical process indicator demonstrating the colour change which occurs when they have been through a sterilization cycle.

left on a radiator, so store under conditions that will not adversely affect the performance of the chemicals, e.g. a cool and dry place.

LOADING THE STERILISER

To sterilise effectively, steam needs to be able to circulate freely. Try to avoid creating trapped air pockets when loading the machine that will prevent the steam making direct contact with the instruments, e.g. place kidney dishes at an angle so that the air is not trapped inside the bowl. Placing items in pouches will create an air envelope around the device, which will lower the temperature on the instrument surface and could lead to sterilization failure. Pouches and wrapping of instruments or trays are therefore only appropriate for vacuum sterilisers which can reproducibly remove trapped air.

Best practice guide: loading the steriliser

- Instruments should be clean and dry prior to sterilization

- Sterilisers should never be overloaded; steam should be able to circulate freely

- Instruments should be placed across the tray ribs and should not be touching

- Hinged instruments should be opened

- Bowls, kidney dishes, etc., should be inverted and placed at an angle to allow draining and the steam to contact all surfaces of the vessel

HOW TO OPERATE THE STERILISER

An outline of the key procedures for operating a vacuum and non-vacuum steriliser in the dental practice is given below.

Best practice guide: summary of key points for operating a steriliser

- Steriliser should be installed and validated by a registered competent person (an engineer proficient in testing sterilisers)

- A schedule should be arranged for periodic testing by a qualified test person, quarterly and/or annually (BS EN ISO 13060)

- A named person in the practice is accountable for the steriliser's validation, periodic testing, maintenance and use

- Operator must be trained

- Non-vacuum steriliser must only be used for its intended purpose (solid and unwrapped instruments)

- Wrapped, tubular and textile items should be processed in vacuum steriliser

- A logbook containing validation, maintenance and periodic test records should be maintained for a minimum of 2 years if instruments are used on children

- Daily checks performed by the owner/user (ACT ± steam penetration test (vacuum steriliser only) are required. Record pass/fail of daily ACT and action taken if cycle fails. Keep a record in the logbook

- Vacuum steriliser: weekly checks consisting of ACT, steam penetration test, air leakage and air detection system function test plus door and pressure vessel safety checks should be performed

- Permanent record of every sterilization cycle (paper or electronic format) should be kept; cycle number of instrument tray in patients notes should be recorded

- Instruments should be cleaned and dried prior to sterilization

- Do not overload with instruments (place inverted, angled, with hinges open); do not allow to touch

- Non-wrapped items should ideally be used directly from the steriliser

- RO or sterile (low-mineral, pathogen- and endotoxin-free) water should be used in the reservoir

- Recycled sterile water in the reservoir must be changed daily or if using RO or distilled water at the end of the session, preferably every 4 hours. Water should not be 'topped up'

- The reservoir should be drained down and emptied at the end of the day. Reservoir should be cleaned, rinsed and dried after draining down according to manufacturer's instructions

- Inside and outside of steriliser should be cleaned regularly with a non-linting cloth

- Weekly safety checks of steriliser's pressure safety systems (e.g. door lock and seal) should be performed

- The door should not be opened while the chamber is pressurised

- Be covered by third-party pressure vessel liability insurance

STORAGE OF WRAPPED AND UNWRAPPED INSTRUMENTS

It is inadvisable to leave instruments in the steriliser overnight as confusion can arise as to whether or not they were processed. In the worst-case scenario, contaminated and non-sterile instruments have inadvertently been used on patients the following day, prompting the necessity for a look-back investigation to check for seroconversion to blood-borne viruses. If instruments are left overnight in the steriliser before they are used, you should check the printout to see when the sterilization cycle was run and examine the process indicator. If there is any doubt, then resterilise the instruments before use.

Storage of unwrapped instruments

After the end of the holding period and sterilising cycle, the steam condenses in the steriliser chamber, so the load will be wet unless the steriliser has a drying cycle. Wet instruments can be used directly from the steriliser (as the water will be sterile). The sterilised load becomes contaminated with atmospheric bacteria as soon as the chamber door is opened; therefore, unwrapped instruments should ideally be used immediately.

Best practice guide: methods of storage of unwrapped instruments

- Sterilised wet instruments should be used immediately

- Sterile instruments that are required for minor oral surgery. Allow instruments to dry in the steriliser before opening the door, after which they should

STERILIZATION AND DISINFECTION
OF DENTAL INSTRUMENTS

be placed on a sterile tray, covered with a sterile drape or sterile lid and used within 3 hours

- To store instruments for later use, leave them to *dry* in the steriliser. Immediately after removal from the steriliser instruments may be wrapped using sealed view packs singly or in trays. Storage for up to 21 days is recommended by HTM 0-05. The instruments will not be sterile but their level of microbial contamination should differ little from those used directly from the steriliser if kept in a clean and dry condition. Microorganisms carried in dust particles in the atmosphere are unlikely to proliferate in dry conditions

Best practice guide: storage of wrapped instruments processed in a vacuum steriliser

- Wrapped instruments processed in a vacuum autoclave with a drying cycle can be stored for up to 6 months (HTM 01-01) in a clean, dry and dust-free environment. Collection of dust on the packaging may compromise its integrity and reduce the shelf life
- If the wrapping or sterilization pouches are wet on removal from the steriliser or subsequently become wet during storage, the contents will no longer be sterile and will require re-sterilization
- Do not attempt to dry damp packages
- Record the date and cycle number on the packaging or pouch
- Use stock rotation based on the instrument date

Instrument traceability

It is important to be able to trace the history of instruments through the decontamination cycle (tracking) and their use on different patients (traceability); achieving this is a major challenge to the profession. Rationalisation of the instruments used during routine clinical procedures into standard sets of instruments simplifies and streamlines the decontamination process. In order to aid instrument traceability, keep sets of instruments together in the trays or cassettes so that the tray rather than the individual instrument is the unit of tracking. Sophisticated tracking systems that can read bar codes laser printed on individual instruments are in use in sterile service departments, but this type of technology is currently inappropriate in a small dental practice with limited stocks of instruments. Trays can be identified by colour coding. Alternatively, peel-off labels printed with an identification number and date of reprocessing are suitable for tray packs and instrument pouches. The label is then placed in the patient's notes.

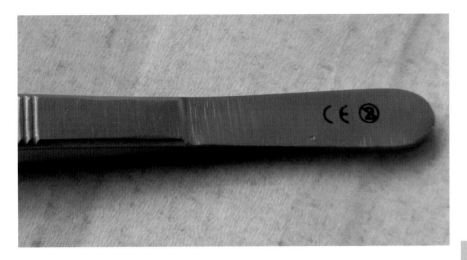

Figure 7.9 International symbol designating 'single-use only' on disposable tweezers. Note the pitting and striations of the metal surface of this single-use item, which would impede any attempts at re-sterilization.

SINGLE-USE ITEMS

> *Never reuse medical devices designated for single use.*

A single-use instrument is a medical device that is intended to be used on an individual patient during a single procedure and then discarded. It should not be reused even on the same patient. Instruments and equipment manufactured for single use carry the symbol of a 2 crossed through with a line (see Figure 7.9).

The reuse of single-use dental equipment can compromise its safety, performance and effectiveness, exposing patients, clinicians or students to unnecessary risk. By definition, single-use devices have not undergone extensive manufacturer testing and validation to ensure that the device is safe to reuse. Reprocessing a single-use device may alter its characteristics so that plastics become brittle or low-grade metals corrode during sterilization. The device may fail mechanically with reuse due to stress fatigue. Single-use devices are often not designed to allow effective decontamination as they have sharp angles, coils or narrow-gauge tubing. Studies have shown that due to the surface defects and pitting of the metal surface of matrix bands, files and reamers, they cannot be successfully decontaminated by cleaning and sterilization. Proteinaceous material which can harbour microbes and prions adheres to the walls of the pits and crevices in the metal surface protected from scrubbing brushes and water jets.

STERILIZATION AND DISINFECTION OF DENTAL INSTRUMENTS

Table 7.5 Categories of dental equipment best replaced with single-use items

- Hard-to-clean items with narrow lumens: saliva ejectors and suction tips
- Brushes: demonstration toothbrushes, rubber prophy cups and bristle brushes
- Complex intricate devices: stainless steel burs, endodontic files, reamers and plastic impression trays
- Invasive instruments and sharps: matrix bands, scalpels, needles and suture needles

Note: The list is not exhaustive; it contains examples only.

If the dentist decides to reuse a single-use item, the product liability for its performance is then transferred from the manufacturer to themselves. This means that the person who reprocesses a single-use device has the same legal obligations and responsibilities under the Medical Devices Regulations as the original manufacturer of the device. If the device after reprocessing is no longer 'fit for the intended purpose' then the dentist may be committing an offence and is at risk of prosecution under both the European and the UK law.

Rationale for single-use items

> *Endodontic files are difficult to clean and should be single use only.*

To avoid the problems associated with reprocessing of hard- or impossible-to-clean and -sterilise instruments such as devices with narrow lumens (e.g. aspirator tips) or brushes, current advice is to replace reusable instruments whenever technically and practically possible with single-use alternatives (Table 7.5). Prompted by concerns over the difficulties associated with removing prion from metal instruments, manufacturers have responded by producing a full range of dental instruments in a single-use disposable format. There is a caveat, important lessons were learnt from the wholesale transference to single-use instruments for tonsillectomies, a procedure considered to be high risk for the transmission of vCJD. Unfortunately, the initial design of single-use instruments did not have the same high-performance specification of the standard instruments and tragically a number of deaths occurred because the instruments failed during surgery. Therefore, single-use instruments must be of high quality and equivalent performance standard as reusable instruments.

The wholesale shift to single-use instruments would not be practical in dentistry because of the high revenues costs of purchasing the instruments plus the increased costs associated with storage and hazardous waste disposal. The additional use of precious raw resources and the high energy consumption involved in disposing of contaminated metal single-use instruments is likely to generate a negative environmental impact. In order to circumvent these problems, some manufactures will collect and then recycle metal instruments for non-medical purposes, but the carbon footprint for reprocessing the waste is still highly significant.

SINGLE-USE INSTRUMENTS AND vCJD

Total number of deaths from vCJD in Europe is approximately 250, the majority of whom (163 cases (figures up to March 2008)) originated from the UK. Human cases of vCJD linked to consuming foods tainted with bovine spongiform encephalopathy (BSE) were first diagnosed in 1995 with the epidemic peaking in 2000 with 6 deaths per quarter in mid-2000, declining to a current incidence of about 1.2 deaths per quarter.

The epidemic of BSE in cattle has been controlled and infected animals removed from the human food chain. Therefore, if successive waves of infection arise, they are likely to be the result of person-to-person spread. In the UK, the National Anonymous Tonsil Archive was established to determine the number of carriers of vCJD in the population. Initial figures published in 2004 based on testing 12 000 tonsils for vCJD found three positive cases. Extrapolation of the figures indicated that approximately 3800 people are incubating the disease in the UK (but the latest projected figures suggest that the figure may be closer to 6000 carriers). Many of these people may remain as long-term asymptomatic infectious carriers of the disease, posing a potential risk for cross-infection to others when they use health care services.

Evidence that vCJD could be transmitted iatrogenically is based on past experience with the sporadic form of Creutzfeldt–Jakob disease (CJD). Infection was transferred to patients receiving contaminated CNS (central nervous system) tissue derived from donors with sporadic CJD. Infected tissue came from several sources including hormones prepared from human pituitary glands, dura mater and corneal grafts. Transmission also followed neurosurgical procedures performed using inadequately decontaminated surgical instruments previously used on patients with CJD.

CJD prions are confined to the CNS, whereas vCJD prions are detected in the CNS and in the peripheral nervous system and lymphoid tissues. Four cases of transmission of vCJD via blood transfusion were reported in 2003–2004 in the UK. Each of the cases had received blood from donors who appeared well at the time of donation, but later died of vCJD. Prions have also been identified in the trigeminal ganglion and tonsils from patients at postmortem.

Armed with this knowledge, we can make an initial risk assessment of the likelihood of prion's transmission occurring during dental treatment. As with all emerging pathogens our knowledge base is in its infancy and continues to evolve as our understanding grows. Abrasion of the lingual tonsil is considered a highly unlikely event during routine dental treatment, but could occur during maxillofacial procedures. Dental pulp, which is composed of vascular and peripheral nerve tissue, was shown in animal studies to be infected with vCJD. Similarly, the dental pulp of individuals sub-clinically infected with vCJD may be infectious, although the level of infectivity is unknown.

Several surveys have shown that most dentists reuse endodontic files and reamers. Appreciable quantities of residual pulp tissue remain adherent to the surface of an endodontic instrument after cleaning and sterilization. A small percentage of endodontic treatments will be carried out on asymptomatic carriers of vCJD. In the UK, over a million endodontic treatments are performed every year. As a result of the large number of treatments, the statistical probability for cross-infection between patients involving contaminated reused endodontic instruments is substantially magnified. As infected carriers move in and out of the dental and medical health care systems, every episode of treatment becomes an opportunity for further transmission of vCJD. A self-sustaining epidemic centred on the health care system could become a reality. Therefore, restricting endodontic files and reamers to single-use only, a stroke eliminates this dental route of transmission and with it the potential for ramifications through the rest of the health service.

DISINFECTION OF HEAT-SENSITIVE EQUIPMENT

In the past, the so-called *cold sterilization* of dental instruments with the disinfectant glutaraldehyde was commonly used in dentistry. Nowadays, most modern dental equipment is manufactured to withstand steam sterilization or is available as a disposable single-use item. So, except for the disinfection of heat-sensitive equipment that cannot be reprocessed by any other method, chemical disinfection is strongly discouraged in dental practice. Glutaraldehyde has gone out of favour as a disinfectant because it is a potent irritant and sensitises the skin, eyes and respiratory tract. Table 7.6 shows the ideal properties for a chemical disinfectant for heat-sensitive dental instruments, dental impressions or hard surfaces (e.g. bracket tables and worktops). Always select a disinfectant that is compatible with the instrument and will not damage the surface or have a deleterious effect on its function. Health and safety legislation requires that a COSHH (Control of Substances Hazardous to Health) assessment is prepared for all disinfectants used in a practice; this is normally derived from the manufacturer's safety data sheet. See Tables 12.2 and 12.3 in Appendix for a description of the types of disinfectants suitable for use in the dental surgery and methods for disinfecting specific items of equipment.

Best practice guide: chemical disinfection of heat-sensitive equipment

- Thoroughly clean instruments and equipment before disinfection as debris and blood can interfere with the antimicrobial action of the disinfectant (see section on manual cleaning of instruments)

Table 7.6 Ideal properties for a general-purpose dental disinfectant

Non-toxic
Non-allergenic
Non-irritant
Not leave a residue
Non-corrosive
Wide range of antimicrobial activity (including killing or destruction of bacterial spores, *Mycobacteria tuberculosis* and viruses including HIV, HCV and HBV)
Short contact time
Not inactivated by organic material
Have a long shelf life
Carry a 'CE' mark and be supplied with a safety data sheet

HIV, human immunodeficiency virus; HCU, hepatitis C virus; HBU, hepatitis B virus.

- Wear appropriate PPE (visor/goggles, mask, heavy duty gloves and plastic apron) when handling disinfectants and work in a well-ventilated room

- Clean and steam sterilise receptacles used for chemical disinfectant solutions

- Make up a fresh solution of disinfectant at the correct concentration (as specified by the manufacturer)

- Disinfect for the recommended contact time (use a timer)

- Completely immerse devices that can be submerged in the disinfectant to ensure contact with all internal and external parts

- Remove instruments from the disinfectant using an aseptic technique

- Rinse thoroughly in sterile water

- Dry using a sterile non-linting cloth

STERILIZATION AND DISINFECTION OF DENTAL INSTRUMENTS

DISINFECTION OF DENTAL IMPRESSIONS

When taking an impression of the teeth or an edentulous ridge the impression material will become contaminated with saliva, blood, oral microorganisms and coughed up respiratory pathogens. Impressions taken on patients with active tuberculosis were found to harbour *Mycobacterium tuberculosis*.

Best practice guide: disinfection of dental impressions

- Cleane and disinfect all impressions before they are sent to the laboratory

- Wear gloves, mask, goggles/face shield

- Thoroughly rinse all impressions in running water to remove all visible signs of contamination

- Choose a disinfectant that is compatible with impression material. Make up a fresh solution or check that the existing solution is within its use by date. Pour the solution into a clean container with a secure lid

- Immerse the impression in the disinfectant for the specified time. Avoid spray disinfectants, which are less effective at penetrating the complex surface of the impression and may create an inhalation risk

- Rinse off the disinfectant with water

Commercially manufactured plastic impression trays are destined for single patient use only and should be disposed of as hazardous clinical waste by the practice or the dental laboratory. Metal impression trays are reusable and should be thoroughly cleaned preferably in a thermal washer disinfector or alternatively in an ultrasonic bath and then steam sterilised.

FURTHER READING

Department of Health. Health Estates and Facilities Division Decontamination (2007). Health Technical Memorandum 01-01: Decontamination of reusable medical devices – Part A (management and the environment). Department of Health's Estates and Facilities Division's Knowledge and Information Portal homepage. Available at http://www.estatesknowledge.dh.gov.uk and http://www.decontamination.gov.uk.

Department of Health. Health Estates and Facilities Division Decontamination (2008). Health Technical Memorandum 01-05: Decontamination in dental facilities. Department of Health's Estates and Facilities Division's Knowledge and Information Portal homepage. Available at http://www.estatesknowledge.dh.gov.uk and http://www.decontamination.gov.uk.

Health Protection Scotland (2005). Local Decontamination Units: Guidance on the Requirements for Equipment, Facilities and Management. NHS National Services Scotland. Available at www.documents.hps.scot.nhs.uk/hai/decontamination/publications/ldu-001-02.pdf.

Health and Safety Executive (2004). Pressure Systems and You. Available at www.hse.gov.uk.

Medicine and Healthcare Regulatory Agency. Device Bulletin (2006). Single-Use Medical Devices: Implications and Consequences of Reuse, 2006 (04). Available at http://www.mhra.gov.uk.

Walker, J.T., Dickinson, J., Sutton, J.M., Raven, N.D.H. and Marsh, P.D. (2007). Cleanability of dental instruments – implications of residual protein and risks from Creutzfeldt–Jakob disease. British Dental Journal, 203, 395–401.

Chapter 8

Dental surgery design, disinfection and managing aerosols

Environmental hygiene is an important component of good infection control and an essential component of standard precautions. Overall, the practice environment should be clean, dry, well lit and well ventilated. This provides not only a pleasant environment to work but also one which increases patient confidence that the practice is a safe and professional surgery to visit.

DENTAL SURGERY DESIGN

Room size

Room should be of sufficient size to allow ready access to dental chair and to perform procedure unhindered (typical size: 17 m^2). The surgery should allow unimpeded access for operators and patients, and have a design which facilitates environmental cleaning, access for disabled and access in case of a medical emergency. (For surgery designs, visit Department of Health Estates and Facilities Directorate (formerly NHS Estates) hosted by the Department of Health website at www.dh.gov.uk.)

Ventilation

Room should be well ventilated (open window) or air conditioned.

- Recommended fresh air supply rate should not be <5–8 L/second per occupant
- Air-cooled air conditioning is preferred; filters should be replaced regularly
- Ventilation systems should exhaust to the outside of the building
- Avoid free-standing or desktop mechanical fans if possible as they circulate dust, splatter and aerosols around the surgery

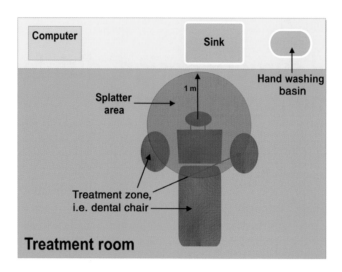

Figure 8.1 Diagram of zones within the dental surgery where contamination is likely to occur.

Work surfaces and zoning

- Areas within clean and dirty 'zones' for practice should be clearly identified to reduce the risk of cross-contamination (Figure 8.1)

- The room should be uncluttered to allow easy access for cleaning

- Work surfaces should be easy to clean, joint free and impermeable, and wherever possible curve up at the wall to avoid sharp, difficult-to-clean corners

Flooring

- Floors should be non-slip and wherever possible curve up the wall by at least 3 inches (to allow effective routine cleaning and cleaning of blood/body fluid spillages)

- The floor should be cleaned daily with detergent and warm water

- Carpets are *not* appropriate as they are harder to keep clean and cannot be reliably disinfected. Bacteria and fungi have been found growing in carpet in surgeries

Dental chair

Dental chair should be impermeable, intact and easy to wipe down. Good chair design with smooth seamless joins in the covering and control panels facilitates rapid cleaning and avoids build-up of microbial contamination.

Lighting

- Lighting should be of a suitable construction that allows easy cleaning and does not allow a build-up of dust

- Lighting used for patient examination must be fitted with a heat filter

- Handles should be covered with disposable plastic cover which is replaced between patients

Fixtures and fittings

- Fixtures and fittings should be clean, and coverings intact and in a good state of repair

- Upholstered furniture should be wipeable. Cloth-upholstered furnishings unless they are specially coated are harder to keep clean and cannot be reliably disinfected

> *Uncoated fabrics are not suitable for use in areas where patient treatment takes place or where contaminated materials are managed (e.g. instrument processing area).*

Washbasins and hand hygiene

- An easily accessible hand washbasin should be available in the room, preferably with elbow-operated mixer taps. It should be specifically dedicated for hand washing and not used for cleaning instruments

- Hand washing sinks should not be fitted with plugs or overflows and the water jet must not flow directly into the plughole

- Wall-mounted (so can be elbow-operated) antimicrobial hand wash solution and non-medicated soap solution (with pump applicator) should be used. Antimicrobial solutions and soaps can become contaminated with microbes and support their growth. Do not top up half-empty containers. Either completely empty, clean and dry containers before refilling or use disposable containers

- Wall-mounted alcohol hand rub/gel should be available for hand decontamination for use on clean hands between patients

- Wall-mounted absorbent disposable paper towels should be provided

Clinical waste

A foot-operated clinical waste sack holder should be conveniently located in the room (see Chapter 10 on clinical waste management).

Sharps containers

An approved sharps container correctly assembled should be located within easy reach of the clinician, but out of the reach of unauthorised persons and children.

Sharps containers should never be placed on the floor.

Storage of equipment and chemicals

- There should be adequate storage to enable the room to remain uncluttered and ensure that work surfaces are readily accessible and easy to clean

- Lockable cupboard(s) should be available to store medicines/disinfectants/ chemicals in accordance with COSHH (1999) regulations

- Sterile stock should be stored on shelving in a secure, cool, dry and clean environment in order to maintain the integrity of the sterile product and its packaging

- Shelving should be readily cleanable and allow for free movement of air around the stored product

Protective clothing

Protective clothing should be readily available in the room, including disposable latex gloves and latex-free alternatives (sterile and non-sterile), disposable plastic aprons, masks and protective eyewear (goggles and visors).

Personal belongings should be kept in a separate room.

Do not eat or drink in the patient treatment area.
Store food in a separate fridge from medicines and dental materials.

SURFACE CLEANING AND DECONTAMINATION

General cleaning

- The practice should have a nominated person to oversee that cleaning standards are maintained. A written protocol may be useful to ensure that standards are maintained

DENTAL SURGERY DESIGN, DISINFECTION AND MANAGING

- All areas should be cleaned and damp dusted regularly. Detergent and hot water are adequate for most routine cleaning requirements. The dental clinical area should be cleaned and damp dusted daily

- Equipment such as mops, buckets and cloths should be specifically designated for the area of use and stored clean and dry. Mops should be washed regularly and stored inverted after use

Surface cleaning

The area around the dental unit becomes contaminated by direct splatter, by droplet nuclei and by touching surfaces with gloved hands. Surface cleaning prevents transmission of infection by direct contact with hands and equipment. (*Note*: Hand hygiene also prevents transmission of surface contaminants.) Dental chair, dental handpiece unit, 3-in-1 syringe handle and hoses, lights, bracket table and cabinets, all will require surface cleaning and disinfection. Try to avoid touching and thereby contaminating drawer handles, pens, computer keyboards and door handles with gloved hands. Pens are a well-recognised vehicle for transmission of MRSA.

Areas within the 'dirty zone', dental chair, dental handpiece unit, lights, bracket table and cabinetry, all will require surface cleaning and disinfection (Table 8.1).

You will need to check with the manufacturer whether the equipment can be cleaned with a detergent and/or disinfected. Commonly used surgery disinfectants are veridical and low residue, such as isopropyl alcohol spray or diluted hypochlorite solution (see Table 12.3 in Appendix).

Table 8.1 Areas requiring decontamination between patients

Dirty zones:
• Bracket table and handle
• Dental handpiece unit, connectors and switches
• Dental chair headrest
• Light handle and switch
• Chair handle controls
• Suction connectors
• Spittoon (outside first and then inside and discard disinfection cloth)

DENTAL SURGERY DESIGN, DISINFECTION AND MANAGING

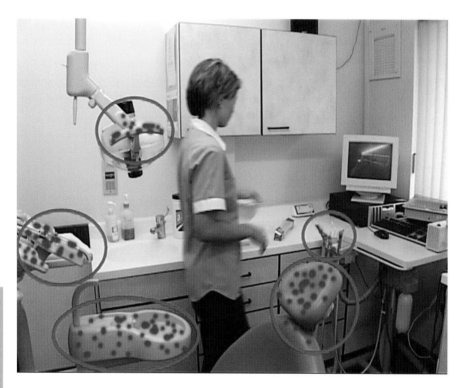

Figure 8.2 Dental surgery showing areas within the 'dirty zone', which require disinfection between patients.

Alcohol wipes are preferred to spray on products because of the generation of unnecessary aerosols, which may cause sensitisation of staff and patients.

Hypochlorite should *not* be used on metal surfaces.

Zoning of work areas

The aim is to separate the areas that are likely to become contaminated by direct contact, aerosols or splatter during treatment procedures ('dirty zones') from those areas unlikely to be directly contaminated ('clean zones'), sometimes referred to as housekeeping surfaces (Recommended Infection Control Practices for Dentistry), (2003). Figure 8.2 shows the areas within the 'dirty zone', which require disinfection between patients.

Zoning is important as it simplifies and increases the efficiency of the decontamination process between patients when time is limited.

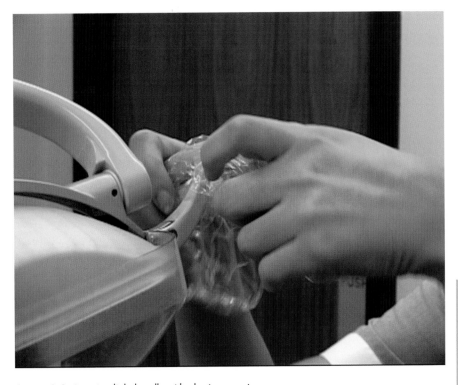

Figure 8.3 Covering light handle with plastic wrapping.

> *Only the 'dirty zones' or visibly soiled areas need to be cleaned and disinfected between each patient, which reduces the time required for decontamination.*

At the end of each clinical session, all work surfaces whether within the clean or dirty zones need to be thoroughly cleaned and disinfected.

Dirty areas which cannot be disinfected easily between patients such as light handle and switches (Figure 8.3), dental unit switches, buttons on 3 in 1, ultrasonic handle, control buttons on the dental chair can be covered with clear plastic wrap (cling film) or plastic sleeves as shown in Figure 8.4. The covering should be disposed of (wearing gloves) into clinical waste containers and replaced between patients. If impermeable plastic coverings are not employed then a surface disinfectant should be used on these items between patients.

The dental chair headrest should be cleaned with a detergent, unless it is visibly soiled with blood or saliva, as repeated use of chemical disinfectants can cause damage to the dental chair. The dental chair manufacturer will recommend a suitable cleaning agent. Key points for zoning and surface cleaning are summarised in Table 8.2.

DENTAL SURGERY DESIGN, DISINFECTION AND MANAGING

Table 8.2 Key points for zoning and surface cleaning

- Dirty zones (likely to be contaminated during dental treatment) should be separated from clean zones

- Clean zones: cabinets, surgery drawers, radiographs and patients' notes, computer keyboards are clean zones and should not be touched with contaminated gloved hands or instruments

- During patient treatment, impervious clinical sheets or plastic sheaves should cover all work surfaces that cannot be readily disinfected between patients

- Items can be passed into 'dirty zones' but contaminated items should not be passed out into 'clean zones'

- Storage containers of dental materials should not be placed in the 'dirty zone'

- Cling film should be removed and 'dirty zones' disinfected between patients

- At the end of a working session, all surfaces should be thoroughly cleaned and disinfected with alcohol spray/wipe or proprietary antimicrobial disinfectant spray/wipe

- Work surfaces should be kept clear overnight

- Trap filters must be removed and cleaned on a regular basis (preferably every night). Should be rinsed thoroughly before being replaced. Bleach or hypochlorite should not be used as they rust metal. Replace according to manufacturer's instructions

---

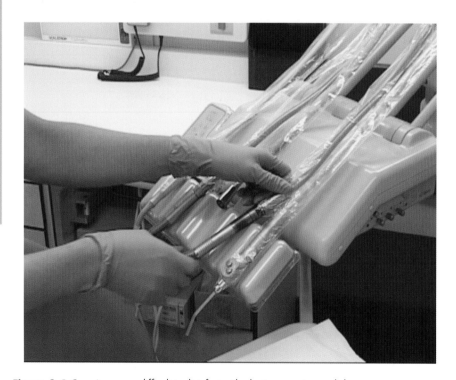

Figure 8.4 Covering areas difficult to disinfect with plastic wrapping and sleeves.

DENTAL SURGERY DESIGN, DISINFECTION AND MANAGING

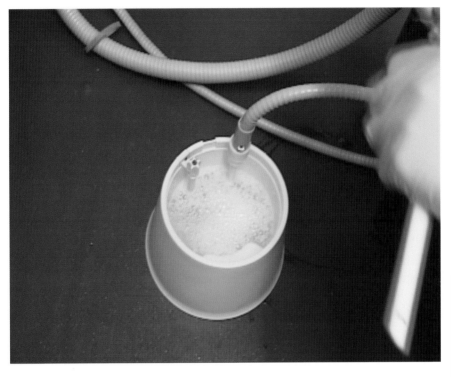

Figure 8.5 Flushing of aspirator suction apparatus with detergent/disinfectant.

Managing aspirators, suction apparatus and spittoons

These require special attention as they become grossly contaminated and are difficult to decontaminate.

- **Spittoons** – clean outer surface first and then inner surface of bowl, add (metered) dose of non-foaming disinfectant, wipe evenly around inside of bowl, leave for time interval specified by manufacturer for disinfectant to destroy microorganisms, rinse with bowl flush and then discard disinfection cloth

- **Aspirators** – flush suction apparatus, drains and spittoons with a non-foaming disinfectant/detergent (e.g. Tridaclens or Orotol) and leave overnight according to the manufacturer's instructions (Figure 8.5)

- **Saliva ejectors** – use them only once as they are hollow tubes which are difficult to clean and sterilise. Single-use ejectors are readily available and cost-effective

> Be careful to avoid back flow from saliva ejectors (high-speed, low-volume aspirators) which are prone to back flow during use and the contents could potentially be expelled into the patient's mouth.

Back flow can happen under the following circumstances:

- If the patient sucks or closes his or her lips around the saliva ejector, pressure in the patient's mouth is less than that in the saliva ejector and a partial vacuum is formed resulting in the back flow of previously aspirated fluids

- When a reversal of pressure is created as the suction tubing is elevated above the patient's mouth. Care should be taken to ensure that the suction tip and line are held below the patient's mouth at all times so that gravity enhances the removal of oral fluids

- When the high-volume suction is switched on in other parts of the suction system in either the same or adjacent surgeries

Fortunately, to date there are no documented cases of infection that have been directly linked to back flow from saliva ejectors. However, members of the dental team should be made aware of the small but potential risk of cross-infection associated with saliva ejectors if they are not handled correctly.

Compressors

Compressed air is used to operate dental chairs, air turbine handpieces, ultrasonic scalers and other equipment in the dental surgery. Oil-lubricated compressors which are the commonest type used in dental practices are prone to colonisation with fungi and pathogenic bacteria. Unless precautions are taken, a small quantity of the lubricating oil, water and bacteria can escape through the oil filters to the airlines and ultimately into the patient's mouth and the surgery environment. Oil contamination of the compressed air compromises the performance of air turbines reducing their longevity and interferes with resin bonding of composite restorations. Dental air needs to be clean and dry. You can minimise the risk of microbial contamination by installing a bacterial filter in addition to a dryer and dust filter. Regularly check the dryness of the dental air supplied to the bacterial filter, as microorganisms can penetrate a bacterial filter if the material becomes wet. You will need to test the quality of the air each year in accordance with manufacturer's instructions. (Further information on the requirements and standards for dental air quality are described in HTM 2022; available at http://www.nhsestates.gov.uk.)

There are legal requirements covering the use of compressors by 'The Pressure Systems Safety Regulations'. Before a compressor is used, a *competent person* must draw up a written scheme which outlines the frequency and extent of examination. Records must be kept to show that examinations have been carried out and the scheme must be reviewed regularly and kept up to date. Air compressors above 250 bar-litres should be examined at least once every 26 months. This requirement is separate from servicing and performance testing.

MANAGEMENT OF AEROSOLS AND SPLATTER

Sneezing, coughing and aerosols generated by rotary instruments produce airborne particles, which vary greatly in size from 0.001 to 10 000 μm. Larger particles or water droplets with a diameter greater than 100 μm are referred to as splatter, which travels through the air for short distances and settles within a radius of 1 m from the source, e.g. patient or basin tap, whereas aerosols consist of smaller ($\leq$10 μm) airborne particles that are capable of remaining in the air for several hours and of travelling long distance on air currents such as into the patient waiting room.

Aerosols are generated by a wide variety of dental procedures including amongst others the use of dental handpieces, ultrasonic instrumentation, orthodontic debonding, and air and water syringing. Coolant dental unit water mixes with blood, saliva, tooth tissue and oral bacteria to produce a contaminated aerosol that can be inhaled into the respiratory passages or deposit on the skin and mucous membranes of the eyes and mouth. Microbes in airborne particulates can be inhaled directly or from particulate debris remaining after the water has evaporated (droplet nuclei). A recent study showed the counts of >1000 cfu/m^2/hour at 1.5-m distance from the patient (Bennett *et al.*, 2000).

Airborne particulates, generated during dental treatment, have been shown (Rautemaa *et al.*, 2006)to decrease to background levels within 10–30 minutes due to the rapid deposition of particles at approximately 1 m from the ground or height of the patient's head (Figure 8.1). Ultrasonic scaling produces the highest concentrations of microbes in the aerosol, with peak concentrations recovered approximately 6–12 inches from the operator.

Aspirators remove approximately 90% of the coolant spray (Figure 8.6). Aspirators should exhaust externally to avoid the spread of potential contamination material within the dental surgery.

Surface cleaning and disinfection remove particulates that have settled out and deposited on equipment and work surfaces. Containment of these aerosols is important; otherwise the 'dirty zone' would potentially have to include the whole room and between-patient decontamination would be impossible. Although there is no evidence to suggest that the bacteria that comprise the normal oral flora pose a serious infectious health risk when aerosolised, respiratory infections including tuberculosis, legionella, SARS (severe acute respiratory syndrome) and flu are spread by aerosols (as discussed

DENTAL SURGERY DESIGN, DISINFECTION AND MANAGING

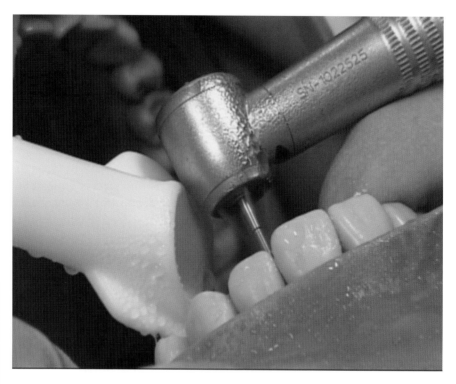

Figure 8.6 Aspirator removing spray generated by air-rotor.

in Chapter 2) and reduction of the risk of occupational infection requires aerosol control and ventilation of the surgery.

Blood can be recovered from saliva samples after many routine dental procedures (e.g. ultrasonic scaling, orthodontic debonding) even if it is not visible to the naked eye. Although it is known that blood-borne pathogens can be transmitted through mucous membrane exposure and blood-born viruses (BBVs) such as human immunodeficiency virus (HIV) and hepatitis B virus (HBV) can be aerosolised during dental procedures; there are no known instances of a blood-borne pathogen being transmitted by an aerosol in a clinical setting. BBVs are transmitted by direct contact following splatter ($\geq$100-μm-size particles) exposure of mucous membranes, although the risk of seroconversion is very much lower than that after a needle-stick injury.

> *Routine use of masks, goggles and visors by dentists, hygienists/therapists and dental nurses will reduce the risks of infection associated with splatter and aerosol.*

Aerosol contamination of the surgery can be minimised by the use of:

- High-volume suction
- Rubber dam

- Proper patient positioning
- Rinsing with chlorhexidine mouth wash prescaling (reduces aerosol contamination for approximately 40 minutes after rinsing)

MANAGING LARGE BLOOD OR BODY FLUID SPILLAGES

Blood and body fluid spillages must be dealt with immediately. The size of the spill (spot, small (<30 mL) or large spill) will determine the management. The majority of blood and body fluid spills in the dental surgery are likely to be spots and splashes. Sodium dichloroisocyanurate (NaDCC) granules or a liquid solution of hypochlorite at 10 000 ppm (1%) should be used for small and large spills, respectively. Disposable gloves, masks and plastic aprons should be worn. (Use eye protection visor/goggles if splashing is likely.) Vomiting may be due to a viral infection, so vomit should be covered immediately with paper towel to prevent aerosolisation and spread of virus particles.

Splashes and spots

- Wear disposable gloves (use masks and plastic aprons if using hypochlorite, and use eye protection visor/goggles if splashing is likely)
- Wipe area with a disposable alcohol wipe or alternatively if the surface is non-porous and compatible with hypochlorite; use a paper towel soaked in diluted hypochlorite (1:100 dilution household bleach)
- If used hypochlorite, then rinse off with clean water to avoid corrosion or bleaching of the surface
- Clean area with water and detergent
- Dry the surface with disposable paper towels
- Discard gloves, alcohol wipes, paper towels as clinical waste
- Wash and dry hands immediately

Small spills (<30 mL)

The use of NaDCC hypochlorite granules (e.g. Haz-tabs granules, Precept) is recommended; if unavailable, follow procedure for large spills outlined below:

- Wear disposable gloves, masks and plastic apron (and use eye protection visor/goggles if splashing is likely)
- Cover spill completely with the granules and wait for the fluid to absorb

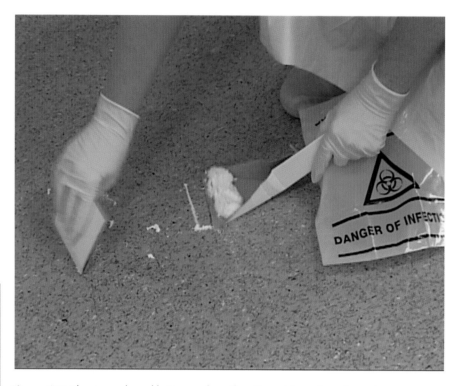

Figure 8.7 Cleaning up hypochlorite granules with a disposable cardboard trowel.

- Leave for 5 minutes

- Collect granules using disposable paper towels and/or cardboard (Figure 8.7). Discard as clinical waste (yellow waste bag)

- Clean area with disposable towels using a fresh hypochlorite solution (1 in 100 dilution) and rinse with clean water as the hypochlorite solution may be corrosive

- Dry the surface with disposable paper towels

- Dispose of towels and protective clothing as clinical waste

- Immediately wash and dry hands thoroughly

Large spills (>30 mL)

Using hypochlorite solution that release 10 000 ppm chlorine (e.g. Haz-tabs, or 1 in 5 dilution of household bleach):

- Wear disposable gloves, masks and plastic apron (and use eye protection visor/goggles if splashing is likely)

- Cover area with disposable towels to limit spread and absorb the liquid

- Pour on freshly prepared hypochlorite solution (1 in 10 dilution household bleach) or prepare solution in accordance with manufacturer's instructions. For Haz-tabs, dissolve one tablet in 250 mL of water to give 10 000 ppm available chlorine or four tablets in 1 L and apply to spill

- Wait for spill to absorb

- Discard towels as clinical waste

- Clean area with disposable paper towels using chlorine solution of 10 000 ppm (or freshly prepared 1 in 100 dilution of household bleach) and rinse with clean water as the hypochlorite solution may be corrosive

- Dry the surface with disposable paper towels

- Dispose of towels and protective clothing as clinical waste

- Immediately wash and dry hands thoroughly

REFERENCES AND WEBSITES

Bennett, A.M., Fulford, M.R., Walker, J.T. *et al.* (2000). Microbial aerosols in general dental practice. *British Dental Journal*, 189, 664–667.

Rautemaa, R., Nordberg, A., Wuolijoki-Saarusti, K. and Meurman, J.H. (2006). Bacterial aerosols in dental practice – a potential hospital infection problem? *Journal of Hospital Infection*, 64, 76–81.

Recommended Infection Control Practices for Dentistry, CDC (2003). Available at http://www.cdc.gov/oralhealth/infectioncontrol/guidelines/index.htm.

Chapter 9

Dental unit waterlines

WHAT ARE BIOFILMS?

Biofilms are complex microbial communities attached to a solid surface and embedded in an organic matrix, which makes them very resistant to removal and penetration by biocides. The biofilms with which dentists are most familiar is dental plaque and it can be appreciated that in that same way that the accumulation of plaques is difficult to control and remove, the control of dental unit waterline (DUWL) biofilms is also challenging to the dental profession.

As the water is continuously moving through the tubes of the working dental unit, how do the microorganisms find enough time to form biofilms? The answer lies in the properties of fluid dynamics and geometry of dental lines (Figure 9.1). A fluid in a tube moves in layers (laminar flow). At the centre of the lumen it travels fastest; the further away from this centre layer the movement becomes slower as a result of friction. Water at the tubing walls is virtually stagnant, allowing bacteria to adhere and colonise the internal surface.

DUWLs are colonised by bacteria derived from the incoming mains water and to a lesser extent by oral bacteria derived from suck-back through the handpiece. In untreated dental units, overnight stagnation and infrequent patterns of use result in amplification of the incoming organisms to form a biofilm on the inner surface of the DUWL (Figure 9.2). This effect is amplified as the DUWL acts as dead leg on the plumbing system. Most dental units are not in active use for an average of 131 hour/week. The DUWL biofilm, like dental plaque, forms rapidly and within a week it can be shedding high bacteria counts of up to 10^{4-6} colony forming units (cfu)/mL into the waterline. Bacteria in biofilms are more resistant to treatment with antimicrobial compounds, ultraviolet light, metal toxicity, acid exposure, dehydration and phagocytosis than corresponding planktonic non-attached cells.

RISK TO STAFF AND PATIENT HEALTH FROM DENTAL UNIT WATERLINES

In the USA and Europe, major outbreaks of waterborne infections affecting, in some instances, thousands of consumers have fuelled widespread public concern regarding the microbiological quality of municipal water supplies. The public's

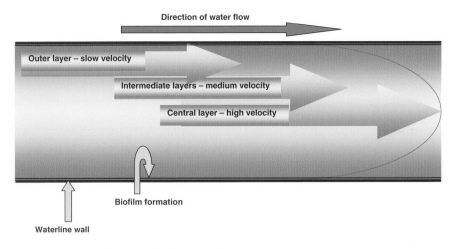

Figure 9.1 Laminar flow in a dental unit waterline.

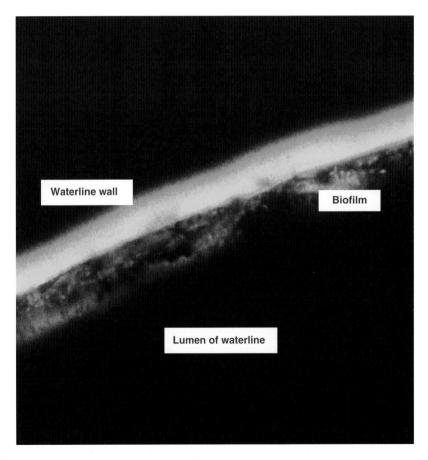

Figure 9.2 Immunofluorescent image of biofilm on dental unit waterlines.

DENTAL UNIT WATERLINES

lack of confidence in water quality is illustrated by an exponential increase in sales of bottled water in many countries, even though the microbiological content of many of these products vastly exceeds that found in tap water. Similar concerns have been expressed over the poor quality of DUWL. The American Dental Association Council on Scientific Affairs stated that contact with water of poor microbial quality is inconsistent with patient expectations of safety and standards of modern dentistry. They set a goal that water used for dental treatment should contain ≤200 cfu/mL of aerobic heterotrophic organism, equivalent to drinking water quality. This figure is somewhat higher than the value set for potable drinking water in Europe of 100 cfu/mL of aerobic heterotrophic organism, but comparable with the department of health HTM 01-05, which stated that the total viable counts should lie in the range of 100–200 cfu/mL, which is considered to be achievable in dental practice in the long-term. This policy has been adopted by other dental governing bodies around the world and has set a challenge for dental equipment manufacturers.

The majority of DUWL contaminants are Gram-negative aerobic environmental species which are non-pathogenic and do not cause infection in immunocompetent people although opportunistic respiratory pathogens, such as *Legionella* spp., *Pseudomonas aeruginosa* and non-tuberculosis *Mycobacterium*, are detected in a proportion of DUWL (Table 9.1). A review of the possible risks to health posed by DUWL had been published in 2007 and these will be considered below (Pankhurst and Coulter, 2007).

Legionellae

Legionellaceae are distributed worldwide in all types of aquatic habitats, generally occurring in low numbers. Legionellae may enter the DUWL from the

Table 9.1 Microorganisms isolated from DUWL

Pseudomonas aeruginosa[a]	*Serratia marcescens*
Burkholderia cepacia[a]	*Nocardia* spp.
Pseudomonas fluorescens	*Streptococcus* spp.
Pseudomonas vesicularis	*Micrococcus* spp.
Pseudomonas posimobilis	*Flavobacterium indologenes*
Pseudomonas pickettii	*Staphylococcus* spp.
Pseudomonas acidovorans	*Staphylococcus saprophyticus*
Pseudomonas testosteroni	*Staphylococcus capitus*
Pseudomonas stutzeri	*Staphylococcus warneri*
Achromobacter xyloxidans	*Legionella* spp.
Xanthomonas maltophilia	*Alcaligenes dentifricans*
Pasteurella haemolitica	*Bacillus* spp.
Pasteurella spp.	*Acinetobacter* spp.
Klebsiella pneumonia	

[a] Important pathogens in cystic fibrosis. (Adapted from Williams *et al.*, 1993; *Journal of American Dental Association*, 124, 59–65.)

mains drinking water and have the ability, under suitable growth and temperature conditions, to multiply and grow in the biofilm to reach the numbers reported between 10^2 and 10^5 cfu/mL. Typical DUWL temperature is 23°C and legionellae proliferate at temperatures between 25 and 42°C. Six to thirty per cent of domestic hot-water systems harbour legionellae and once established can persist for years. The reported prevalence of legionellae in DUWL varies widely from 0 to 68% depending, in part, on the isolation procedures. Variations in recovery rates of *Legionella pneumophila* type 1 are observed with different geographic locations (8% in the USA, 21.8% in Italy and 25% in London), presence of large cold-water tanks and complex plumbing systems, thermal conditions and the type of dental equipment.

Transmission of infection occurs via inhalation of contaminated aerosol droplet, inhalation or rarely aspiration of contaminated water by susceptible individuals. There is no evidence of case-to-case transmission. Legionellosis can present either as an atypical pneumonia or as a milder flu-like illness, known as Pontiac fever.

There is a potential for occupational risk to the dental team and to vulnerable patients (Table 9.2) from exposure to contaminated DUWL aerosols.

Fortunately, the health risks associated with inhaling contaminated DUWL aerosols are thought to be exceedingly low in healthy individuals and there is no published evidence indicating that a patient has ever contracted Legionnaires' disease in a dental chair. The UK national surveillance data found no association between dental treatment and Legionnaires' disease. But there is no room for complacency as a dentist in the USA died from Legionnaires' disease as a result of exposure to legionellae in his surgery's DUWL.

Pseudomonas

Pseudomonads and related species are the predominant bacterial genera found in DUWL and have been isolated from up to 50% of DUWLs. Some of

Table 9.2 Patients at increased risk of Legionnaires' disease

- Existing respiratory disease that makes the lungs more vulnerable to infection
- Illnesses and conditions, such as cancer, diabetes, kidney disease or alcoholism, which weaken the natural defences
- Smoking, particularly heavy cigarette smoking which compromises lung function
- Increasing age, particularly above 50 years
- Sex; males are three times more likely to be infected than females
- Patients on immunosuppressant drugs

DENTAL UNIT WATERLINES

the species in the genera behave as opportunistic pathogens. *P. aeruginosa* accounts for 9–11% of reported nosocomial infections per annum in the USA and Europe, particularly affecting the immunocompromised, those on ventilators, burns patients and patients suffering from cystic fibrosis. The organism can thrive in low-nutrient environments such as distilled water. The latter is commonly employed by dentists as the water for DUWL reservoirs and steriliser reservoirs. Furthermore, pseudomonads grow readily in dilute disinfectants such as chlorhexidine and iodophors and express resistance to a wide range of antibiotics. *P. aeruginosa* is a common coloniser of DUWL and has been isolated from up to 50% of DUWL.

The infective dose for *P. aeruginosa* colonisation in health human volunteers is $>1.5 \times 10^6$ cfu/mL; therefore, the risk for a healthy person becoming colonised following exposure during dental treatment is vanishingly low. There is no direct evidence of *Pseudomonas* infection from a DUWL apart form a single study which showed that two cancer patients were infected by a particular strain of *P. aeruginosa* and 78 non-compromised patients treated in *P. aeruginosa* contaminated dental units were transiently colonised for 3–5 weeks with *P. aeruginosa*, but with no infection, from the dental unit water (Martin, 1987).

Cystic fibrosis patients are at increased risk of infection with *P. aeruginosa* from the DUWL. A recent study concluded that there was only a small risk for cystic fibrosis patients of acquiring *P. aeruginosa* from a dental treatment and the acquisition rate was comparable with the background rate of 1–2% for new infections. However, they caution that the accumulated risk of acquisition associated with frequent dental visits may increase the transmission rate to a clinically significant level.

Mycobacterium

Environmental mycobacterium, i.e. non-tuberculous mycobacterium (NTM), has been shown to proliferate in the dental biofilm. The colony count of non-tuberculous mycobacterium in DUWL exceeded that of drinking water by a factor of 400. Thus, there is a potential risk for large numbers of NTM to be swallowed, inhaled or alternatively inoculated into oral wounds during dental treatment, leading to colonisation and infection. Patients such as those with AIDS are highly susceptible to opportunistic NTM. Identical strains of *Mycobacterium avium* have been isolated from infected AIDS patients and their home cold-water tap for drinking. Fortunately, most NTM infection is asymptomatic as studies suggest that approximately 12% of the population in the USA have been colonised by the NTM (*M. avium*). A small number of cases of NTM infection have been associated directly with dental treatment and it is therefore prudent to reduce contamination by good DUWL management.

Endotoxin

Although no clinical cases of environmental bacterial infections except those due to *P. aeruginosa* have been directly associated with dental procedures, the bacterial cell wall of Gram-negative bacteria is a potent source of endotoxin. Endotoxin can cause localised inflammation, fever and shock. A high bacterial load in the DUWL usually equates with a high endotoxin concentration. A consequence of indoor endotoxin exposure is the triggering or exacerbation of asthma (Pankhurst *et al.*, 2005). Data from a single-large practice-based cross-sectional study reported a temporal association between occupational exposure to contaminated DUWL with aerobic counts of >200 cfu/mL at $37°C$ and development of asthma in the subgroup of dentists in whom asthma arose following the commencement of dental training. USA Pharmacopoeia sets a limit for endotoxin for irrigation sterile water of 0.25 endotoxin units/mL. Endotoxin has been detected in dental water up to 500–2560 units/mL.

METHODS TO REDUCE THE BIOFILM

DUWL management guidelines and commercially available decontamination systems are specifically designed to reduce and maintain environmental Gram-negative aerobic bacteria at an acceptable level ($\leq$200 cfu/mL) in the DUWL. A variety of different methods and commercially available products can be used to improve the quality of water issuing from the DUWL. The main types and methods are outlined below:

> *Dental units should be drained down and waterlines cleaned at the end of each working day.*

Draining down the unit prevents the biofilm from growing during the stagnant period overnight. It is important to prevent the development of the biofilm as it is difficult to remove once established.

> *Waterlines should be flushed for 2 minutes at the start of the day and for 20–30 seconds between patients.*

Flushing reduces the bacterial count by approximately 97%, but will not reduce the total count to $\leq$200 cfu/mL; nor will it remove the biofilm. So, in most units flushing is insufficient on its own to control the bacterial count in the DUWL. In dental units, which are not drained down at night, flushing at

DENTAL UNIT WATERLINES

the start of the day will reduce the bacterial load caused by overnight water stagnation. Flushing between patients helps to prevent cross-contamination by removing oral fluids introduced into the DUWL via suck-back through the handpieces.

> *Antiretraction valves should be fitted to handpieces.*

Antiretraction valves are fitted on modern handpieces or the waterline to reduce suck-back from the oral cavity. An estimated 1 mL of microbe-laden oral fluid can be aspirated into the DUWL if antiretraction valves have not been fitted.

> *Dental unit waterlines must be disinfected daily or weekly.*

Regular, daily or weekly disinfection of the waterlines according to the manufacturer's instructions with products containing one of the following active agents will produce water of drinking water standard (Table 9.3).

A large multicentre European study found that the peroxide-based Dentosep and Oxygenol were the most effective and that continuous applied products performed better than the intermittent applied products (Schel *et al.*, 2006).

Not all products completely remove the biofilm, so regular dosing according to the manufacturer's instructions is required to control the bacterial count. The disinfectant can be introduced with a pressurised pump system or via an independent bottled water system. Some units are fitted with automated continuous dosing systems. Only use a disinfectant that is recommended as compatible with your particular dental unit as unsuitable products can damage internal components resulting in leaks.

Table 9.3 Chemicals used in disinfection of DUWL (examples only the list is not exhaustive)

Hydrogen peroxide (e.g. Dentosept, Oxygenol, Sterilex ultra)
Hydrogen peroxide and silver ions (e.g. Sanosil)
Citric acid (e.g. Alpron)
Chlorhexidine (e.g. Bio Blue)
Electrochemically activated water (e.g. Sterilox)
Peracetic acid (e.g. Dialox)
UV, ozone, iodine, chlorine dioxide, sodium hypochlorite or alcohol

See also Table 12.3 in Appendix.

There is evidence, reviewed by Coleman *et al.* (2007), that disinfectants may produce adverse effects which we should be aware of when deciding on a given product:

- Electrochemically activated oxidising solution: some products may cause degradation of silicone tubing resulting in leakage

- Chlorhexidine-containing products: some products reduce strength of dentine-bonding agents

- Stabilised hydrogen peroxide: some powder-based products associated with clogging of waterlines

- Citric acid-based products: some products may cause leaching of copper components

- Hypochlorite/chlorine: may react with biofilm to produce carcinogenic tri-halomethanes that are associated with an excess risk of rectal/bladder cancer in men

> *Independent bottled water reservoirs are recommended but should not be filled with water from the surgery tap.*

Independent bottled water systems are either integral part of the dental chair or can be installed separately (Figure 9.3). The main advantage is that they

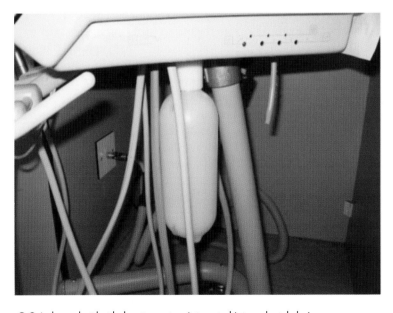

Figure 9.3 Independent bottled water system integrated into a dental chair.

DENTAL UNIT WATERLINES

draw fluids from the bottled reservoir holding sterile or distilled water, or alternatively a dilute biocide aqueous solution, and bypass the municipal water supply, thus avoiding contamination with *Legionella* spp. and other waterborne respiratory pathogens. However, such systems alone cannot reliably improve the quality of treatment water as biofilms are able to form within the bottles unless carefully managed.

Regular cleaning of the inside of the bottles and flushing of the waterlines with a disinfectant is required to reduce adherent microbial biofilms.

Best practice guide: disinfecting waterline reservoir bottles and lines

- At the end of the working day, drain down the water from the waterlines

- Disinfect reservoir bottle with diluted 1:10 (approximately 0.5%) household bleach solution or with the approximately equivalent 5000 ppm solution of Haz-tabs or Precept or with a commercial product (e.g. Alpron, Dentisept, Sterilex Ultra, Bio Blue or Sterilox)

- Rinse with sterile water and store dry and inverted overnight. This will prevent biofilm formation in both the bottle and the waterlines

> Prevent contamination of the mains water supply using a physical air gap and of the dental waterline using point of use filters.

European Union regulations state that there should be a physical gap or *type A air gap* separating the DUWLs from the mains water supply in order to prevent back-siphonage of clinical material into the municipal supply. Compliance can be achieved either by installing a storage tank fitted with water piping with a regulation air gap or by an independent bottled water system to supply water directly to the DUWLs and handpieces.

Disposable microbial filters placed as close as possible to the handpiece will prevent suspended bacteria entering the handpiece, but do not remove the biofilm. These devices used according to manufacturer's instructions can produce dental unit water of drinking water standard or better (Table 9.4).

Table 9.4 Key recommendations to maintain the quality of DUWL and provide potable water

- All waterlines and airlines should be fitted with antiretraction valves

- A bottled water system should be used to supply the dental waterlines

- Disinfectants should be used in the bottle and waterlines (applied according to manufacturer's instructions)

- Regulations for a physical air gap on dental equipment should be followed to prevent back-siphonage

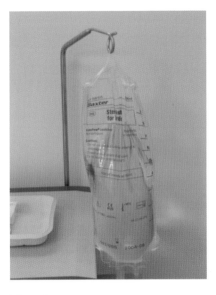

Figure 9.4 Sterile saline delivery bag.

Use sterile water for implant, periodontal and oral surgical irrigation.

Sterile water delivered in a separate delivery system is required for minor oral surgery (MOS) procedures, periodontal and implant surgery (Figure 9.4). The use of sterile or distilled water per se is of no use in solving this problem if it is used within the dental lines already contaminated with a biofilm. For MOS procedures, the guidance from both BDA (British Dental Association) and ADA (American Dental Association) is to irrigate with sterile water or saline. Importantly, for these sterile solutions to remain uncontaminated they need to be delivered through devices other than the DUWL. A variety of delivery systems are commercially available incorporating pump and bagged sterile solutions or fully autoclavable assemblies of reservoirs and handpiece tubing to be used with sterile water (Figure 9.4). The disadvantage of these system is that they can be expensive to purchase and more cumbersome and often less convenient to use than conventional delivery systems. Although when small volumes are required a sterile disposable syringe filled with saline is a suitable alternative.

CONTROL OF LEGIONELLAE IN DENTAL UNIT WATERLINES

Since dentists provide water which may potentially have health consequences for the public, there is a legal requirement for dentist to control the Legionella bacteria in their water systems. In order to comply with their legal duties,

DENTAL UNIT WATERLINES

Table 9.5 Thermal control of Legionellae

Hot-water plumbing

● Storage of water should be avoided between 20 and 45°C

● Hot water should be stored at 60°C

● Aim is to achieve hot water at 50°C at all points of use within 1 minute of turning on the hot tap. To avoid scalds; use hazard notice stating, 'Be careful very hot water'. Infrequently used taps should be flushed for several minutes on a weekly basis

Cold-water plumbing

● Cold water tanks should be sited in a cool place and thermally insulated

● The amount of water stored should be kept to a minimum and be equivalent to one day's usage

● The water temperature should be below 20°C after running the taps for 2 minutes

Recommended monitoring and recording

● Temperature of sentinel hot and cold taps should be checked monthly

● Biannual monitoring should be done to ensure that the incoming cold water to the premises is below 20°C at the ball valve outlet of the cold-water storage tank

● There should be an annual visual inspection of the tanks with cleaning and disinfection as required

● If taste and odour problems are noted then a microbiological investigation may be required as this could signal development of conditions that could promote growth of legionellae

Based on HSC (2000).

DENTAL UNIT WATERLINES

dentists should identify and assess sources of risk that are likely to encourage the organisms found in DUWL and dental surgery plumbing to multiply and become aerosolised. They should prepare a scheme for preventing and controlling the risk. A brief summary of the key advice in guidelines pertaining to dental practice is outlined in Table 9.5. (For a full explanation of the guidelines, please consult the Code of Practice, which is available from HSE books available on http://www.tsoshop.co.uk/ and on the web from the Health Protection Agency at http://www.hpa.org.uk/infections/topics_az/legionella/advice.htm and Water Systems Health Technical Memorandum 04-01.)

REFERENCES AND WEBSITES

Pankhurst, C.L. and Coulter, W.A. (2007). Do contaminated dental unit waterlines pose a risk of infection? *Journal of Dentistry*, 35, 712–720.

Martin, M.V. (1987). The significance of the bacterial contamination of dental unit water systems. *British Dental Journal*, 163, 152–154.

Pankhurst, C.L., Coulter, W.A., Philpott-Howard, J.J. *et al.* (2005). Evaluation of potential risk of occupational asthma in dentist exposed to contaminated dental unit water lines. *Primary Dental Care*, 12, 53–59.

Schel, A.J., Marsh, P.D., Bradshaw, D.J. *et al.* (2006). Comparison of the efficacies of disinfectants to control microbial contamination in dental unit water systems in general dental practices across the European Union. *Applied and Environmental Microbiology*, *73*, 1380–1387.

Coleman, D.C., O'Donnell, M.J., Shore, A.C. *et al.* (2007). The role of manufacturers in reducing biofilms in dental chair waterlines. *Journal of Dentistry*, *35*, 701–711.

HSC (2000). *The Control of Legionella Bacteria in Water Systems. Approved Code of Practice and Guidance.* ISBN 0-7176-1772-6. Available at http://www.tsoshop.co.uk/.

FURTHER READING

Pankhurst, C.L. (2006). BDA Fact File. Contaminated Dental Unit Waterlines. Available at http://www.bda.org.uk.

Advice on Legionella available from Health Protection Agency, United Kingdom. Available at http://www.hpa.org.uk/infections/topics_az/legionella/advice.htm.

Water Systems Health Technical Memorandum 04-01: The Control of Legionella, Hygiene, 'Safe' Hot Water, Cold Water and Drinking Water Systems. Available at http:// www.tsoshop.co.uk/.

DENTAL UNIT WATERLINES

Chapter 10

Health care waste management

LEGISLATION ON HAZARDOUS WASTE DISPOSAL

The primary message in all European Union waste management strategies is to manage waste sustainably by:

- Reducing the volume of waste produced per capita
- Limiting the number of landfill sites
- Protecting the environment from pollution by hazardous effluents

This 'green' approach to clinical waste is reflected in national legislation (Hazardous Waste Regulations 2005 and List of Waste Regulations 2005). Under the current regulations, the dentist and the dental practice is defined as a waste 'producer'. The dentist, therefore, has full responsibility and a duty of care for ensuring that waste is segregated, transported and disposed of according to national and international guidelines. As an employer, the dentist is responsible for protecting all members of their dental team, patients and waste disposal contractors from accidental exposure to hazardous waste. All members of the dental team can make a contribution to protecting the environment by reducing the amount of unnecessary waste and recycling waste whenever possible.

On a practical level, each dental practice is required to prepare its own waste policy and to identify which member(s) of the staff are responsible for overseeing the local management of health care waste including:

- Segregation of hazardous from non-hazardous waste streams
- Handling and on-site storage
- Waste collection
- Record keeping

Fortunately, in the UK, the dentist is guided through this complex web of legislation by a code of practice entitled 'Environment and Sustainability HTM 07-01: Safe Management of Health Care Waste – 2006'. The key features of the code of practice are outlined in Box 10.1.

> **Box 10.1** Key features from the code of practice (HTM 07-01 – 2006) on premises notification and disposal of health care waste
>
> - The regulator (Environment Agency in the UK) has adopted a 'unified' approach for consigning hazardous infectious and medicinal waste that is complicit with the health and safety, transport and waste regulations
> - Dentists as producers of health care waste have a duty of care to ensure that all health care waste is managed and disposed of properly
> - It is a legal requirement in England and Wales for waste producers to segregate hazardous and non-hazardous waste at source since it is no longer permissible to dispose of hazardous and non-hazardous material at the same landfill site
> - Transfer and consignment notes must contain a written description of the waste and the appropriate EWC codes
> - Producers (consignors) of hazardous waste must notify their premises to the Environment Agency[a]. A dental premise is exempted from notification if it produces <200 kg of hazardous waste material per year (which includes hazardous non-clinical items such as fridges, TVs, computer screens) and the hazardous waste is removed from the premises by a registered carrier
> - Movement of hazardous waste from premises that are not either notified (registered) or exempted is prohibited; in doing so a criminal offence is committed
> - Each dental premise producing waste is assigned a unique six-digit premise reference code that is used to identify and track the movement of the waste
> - Owners of multiple practices are required to register each practice separately
> - The producer must ensure that the waste falls within the terms of the waste contractor's waste management licence, permit or exemption
> - The producer must keep transfer notes from the waste carrier for 2 years and consignment notes and returns from waste disposal contractor for 3 years

Modified from Code of Practice 'Environment and sustainability HTM 07-01: Safe management of health care waste – 2006'.
EWC, European waste catalogue.
[a] In Northern Ireland, the waste producer must pre-notify the Environment and Heritage service prior to each collection and movement of hazardous waste. In England and Wales, dental premises are registered with the regulator on annual basis.

TYPES OF WASTE

Most dental practices will generate four main types of waste (see Figure 10.1):

- Clinical waste
- Medicines waste

- 'Offensive' waste
- Trade waste

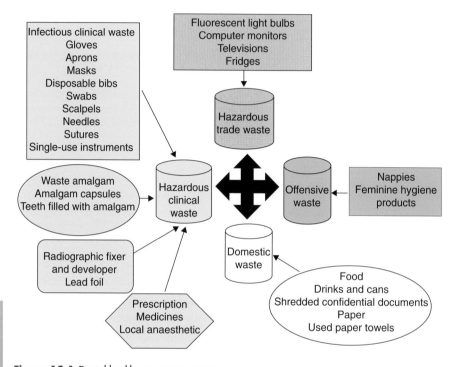

Figure 10.1 Dental health care waste streams.

The remainder of this chapter will focus on the disposal of waste generated by clinical treatment. For information on the disposal of trade and domestic waste or recycling, please refer to the Department for Environment, Food, and Rural Affairs and Environment Agency websites listed at the end of the chapter.

WHAT IS HAZARDOUS WASTE?

Not all clinical waste is hazardous waste.

A hazardous waste is a waste with one or more properties that are hazardous to health or the environment, e.g. explosive, oxidising, highly flammable, flammable, irritant, infectious, toxic, carcinogenic, teratogenic, mutagenic, harmful, toxic gases and ecotoxic.

> **Box 10.2** Clinical waste (according to the Controlled Waste Regulations 1992) is any waste which consists wholly or partly of:
>
> - Human or animal tissue
> - Blood or bodily fluid
> - Excretions
> - Drugs or other pharmaceutical products
> - Swabs or dressings
> - Syringes, needles or other sharp instruments
> - Any other waste arising from dentistry which may cause infection or unless rendered safe may prove hazardous to any person coming into contact with it

Clinical waste as defined in Box 10.2 is categorised as a hazardous waste. Prior to disposal in landfill sites, the traditional method for reducing the volume and mass of clinical waste and making it safe has been incinerated. But a burgeoning body of evidence has questioned the efficacy and safety of incineration. Of particular concern is pollution from exhaust emissions, especially when incinerators are located in residential or environmentally sensitive areas. For instance, viable bacteria can be released from exhaust flues under certain circumstances. Temperature gradients form in the incinerator exhaust stack and pathogenic bacteria can survive in the cooler zones at the base of the stack. These and similar concerns have prompted the introduction of more reliable and environment-friendly disinfection methods referred to collectively as 'alternative technology methods' which employ heat, chemicals or irradiation.

Heat processes can be divided into high- and low-temperature methods (Figures 10.2 and 10.3).

All of these processes are intended to render the waste non-hazardous, unrecognisable and acceptable for landfill. In general, alternative technology methods operate at lower temperatures than those generated during incineration. For example, microwaving exposes the waste to temperatures in the range of 95–98°C and is deemed unsuitable for wastes containing metal objects, body parts, toxic chemicals and radioactive substances. So, it is essential that the waste disposal contractor is made aware of the exact contents of the sharps receptacle (bin) so that the waste is treated using the appropriate process. Approximately, 95% of clinical waste produced in hospitals can be effectively treated with alternative technology processes. Notable exceptions include infectious waste containing Variant Creutzfeldt–Jakob disease, cytotoxic medicines, large metallic objects and anatomical waste which will require incineration. Once a waste is rendered free of infection using any of these methods, then it is no longer considered to be hazardous.

HEALTH CARE WASTE MANAGEMENT

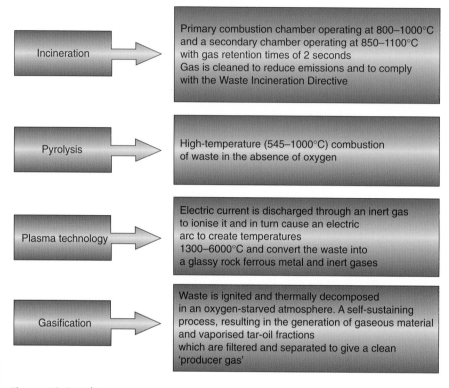

Figure 10.2 High-temperature processes.

HAZARDOUS WASTE REGULATIONS AND THE EUROPEAN WASTE CATALOGUE CODE

All waste must be segregated according to its European waste catalogue code.

According to the Hazardous Waste Regulations 2005, the dentist is legally obliged to segregate and consign, i.e. label waste for collection with a brief written description of the waste and the appropriate EWC (European waste catalogue) code. Developed by the European Commission and applicable across all the states of the European Union, the EWC (2002) code classifies individual waste products under 20 main chapter headings that are linked to an industrial sector. Each type of waste product is assigned a six-digit code. Hazardous waste is marked with asterisk (*) after the code number. The chapters applicable to dental health care waste are Chapter 18 of the EWC for the waste from natal care, diagnosis, treatment or prevention of diseases in humans (see Table 10.1) and Chapters 9 and 15 of the EWC for the consignment of X-ray fixer and developer.

HEALTH CARE WASTE MANAGEMENT

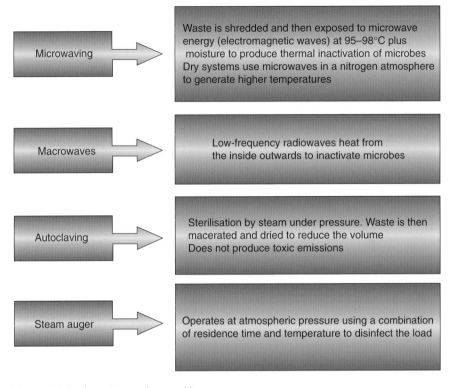

Figure 10.3 Alternative non-burn and low-temperature processes.

Infectious clinical waste

According to the guidance set down in the code of practice, the dentist would be expected to perform a task-based risk assessment to decide whether or not an item of waste is hazardous. Much of the clinical waste produced from patient's treatment is contaminated with blood or saliva, and hence is potentially infectious. In order to assess the potential risk of infection, the following legal definition for infectious waste is applied:

> "*Substances containing viable microorganisms or their toxins which are known or reliably believed to cause disease in man or other living organisms.*"

Note that even minor infections are included within the definition of infectious waste. However, insufficient information may be known about the health and blood-borne virus carrier status of the patient to make an informed decision. On behalf of the dental profession, the regulatory authority has decided to interpret the definition of infectious waste in line with standard precautions for infection control (see Chapter 2), whereby all clinical waste contaminated with blood or other body fluids such as saliva are to be consigned and labelled as

Table 10.1 EWC codes for use in dental practice

Chapters 9 and 15 of EWC

- 09 01 03* Solvent-based developer solutions

- 09 01 04* Fixer solutions

- 15 01 10* Packaging containing residues of or contaminated by dangerous substances (i.e. lead foil)

Chapter 18 of EWC

Waste from natal care, diagnosis, treatment or prevention of diseases in humans

- 18 01 01   Sharps except 18 01 03*

- 18 01 02   Body parts and organs including blood bags and blood preserves (except 18 01 03*)

- 18 01 03* Waste whose collection and disposal is subject to special requirements in order to prevent infection

- 18 01 04   Waste whose collection and disposal is not subject to special requirements in order to prevent infection, e.g. dressings, plaster casts, linen, disposable clothing

- 18 01 06* Chemicals consisting of dangerous substances

- 18 01 07   Chemicals other than those listed in 18 01 06*

- 18 01 08* Cytotoxic and cytostatic medicines

- 18 01 09   Medicines other than those mentioned in 18 01 08*

- 18 01 10* Amalgam waste from dental care

---

*Refers to hazardous waste regardless of threshold concentration.

18 01 03 infectious hazardous waste, e.g. used gloves, masks, plastic aprons etc. Excluded from the definition are items such as disposable paper towels used for drying washed hands, which are non-hazardous and can be segregated for recycling with other paper waste.

Anatomical waste and teeth

> Never incinerate amalgam waste because it releases toxic mercury compounds.

Recognisable body parts (surgical specimens) are considered to be offensive to the general public and must be disposed in yellow receptacles or bags and incinerated. Teeth do not fall into this category as they are not considered to offend the sensibilities of the public and therefore do not require incineration. Dispose extracted teeth in the infectious sharps waste. Teeth-containing amalgam must never be incinerated or disposed of using alternative technology methods as toxic mercury compounds are released into the atmosphere by these processes. Instead, they should be segregated from other health care waste. Store them in a white-lidded rigid container containing a mercury suppressant, prior to appropriate recovery/disposal of the amalgam by a licenced specialist waste disposal contractor.

Classification of prescription-only medicines waste

Medicines fall into three categories:

1. Cytotoxic and cytostatic (not used in routine dental treatment)

2. Pharmaceutically active, but not cytotoxic and cytostatic (e.g. local anaesthetic solution)

3. Not pharmaceutically active and possessing no hazardous properties (examples include saline (e.g. used as an irrigant) and glucose

Only cytotoxic or cytostatic medicines, i.e. possessing hazardous characteristics, such as toxic, carcinogenic, teratogenic or mutagenic, are now classified as hazardous waste. Current recommendations are based on the descriptions published in the British National Formulary, National Institute for Occupational Safety and World Health Organization. Medicinal waste includes expired, unused, spilt, contaminated pharmaceutical products, drugs, vaccines and sera. The category also includes discarded items used in the handling of pharmaceuticals, such as packaging contaminated with residues, gloves, masks, connecting tubing, syringe bodies and drug vials. This is interpreted to include partially discharged local anaesthetic cartridges which should be disposed of as medicinal waste. However, regardless of their classification, the disposal route for POM (prescription-only medicine) waste has not changed and remains incinerate at a suitably authorised facility. This is because POM cannot be sufficiently degraded by low-temperature alternative technologies, e.g. microwaving, and therefore require incineration. In England and Wales, it is a legal requirement of the Hazardous Waste Regulations to segregate infectious and medicinal waste. Practices are required to have two puncture-proof sharps bins in the surgery for the disposal of:

- Infectious waste and fully discharged sharps (orange lid) (Figure 10.4)

- POM waste, e.g. partially discharged local anaesthetic cartridges and needles (yellow lid) (see Table 10.2)

HEALTH CARE WASTE MANAGEMENT

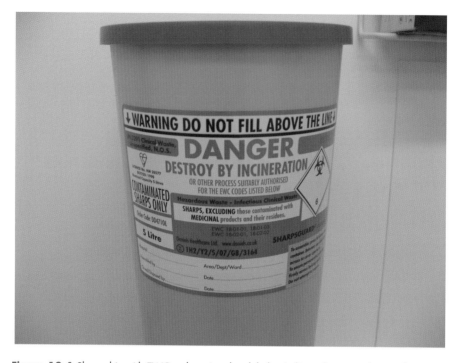

Figure 10.4 Sharps bin with EWC codes printed on label to indicate the types of waste that can be disposed of in an orange-lidded bin.

Radiographic fixer and developer solutions and lead foil from radiograph packets are classified as hazardous. These hazardous wastes should be stored in a leakproof container before collection by a suitably licenced waste contractor for either recovery or disposal.

AMALGAM WASTE AND INSTALLATION OF AMALGAM SEPARATORS

> Amalgam waste must be removed using an amalgam separator and disposed of as a hazardous waste.

The main impact on the dental profession of the waste regulations is the disposal of amalgam, which is now classified as a hazardous waste with its own EWC code (18 01 10). In practical terms, this means that the surgery must segregate all forms of waste amalgam from other waste streams and prevent amalgam entering the waste water system.

HEALTH CARE WASTE MANAGEMENT

Table 10.2 Colour code denotes identification, segregation and method of waste disposal

Colour code	Type of waste	Mode of treatment and disposal
Black or clear waste sacks	Domestic; non-hazardous trade waste, e.g. paper	Landfill or recycling
Orange-lidded sharps bins	Infectious sharps	Alternative treatment plant or incineration
	Teeth not filled with amalgam	
	Fully discharged sharps contaminated with non-cytotoxic medicines	
Orange waste sacks	Hazardous infectious clinical waste, e.g. swabs, used gloves, masks, plastic aprons, disposable gowns	Alternative treatment plant or incineration
Yellow-lidded sharps bins	Non-cytotoxic medicinal waste including partially discharged or unused local anaesthetic cartridges	Incineration
Yellow waste sacks	Anatomical waste	Incineration
Yellow and black waste sacks	Non-infectious 'offensive waste stream' e.g. nappies, feminine hygiene products	Must be suitably packaged but does not require any treatment prior to deep landfill
White-lidded receptacles	Amalgam waste	Recovery of mercury
Purple-lidded sharps receptacles	Cytotoxic and cytostatic medicines waste and products from preparation	Incineration
Purple waste sacks	Products from preparation of cytotoxic and cytostatic medicines waste	Incineration

Mercury in the environment

Dentistry's contribution to the levels of mercury in the natural environment is negligible. Amalgamation of mercury for dental restorations produces a stable compound that does not readily convert to methyl mercury, the form absorbed by fish. It is methylated mercury that enters the food chain with detrimental, toxic consequences to human health and that of other species. Nevertheless, dentists are obliged to do all they can to protect the environment from mercury. Waste amalgam or amalgam capsules must never be disposed of with other types of clinical waste or poured down the sink. Solid amalgam waste awaiting collection should be stored in white-lidded rigid containers under a mercury

HEALTH CARE WASTE MANAGEMENT

suppressant. Amalgam aspirated from the mouth is removed by an amalgam separator in the waste line of the suction apparatus to stop amalgam entering the drains (waste water system) or sewers.

Fitting of amalgam separators

Chairside traps and vacuum filters are adequate for trapping large particles of debris, but are not fine enough to remove small suspensions of mercury particles. Hence, simple filters and gauzes are no longer compliant with the regulations and are superceded by amalgam separators that meet the BS EN ISO 11143:2000 standard. Amalgam separators operate using one or more of the following technologies: sedimentation, fine filtration, centrifugal force and ion exchange. Separators can be retrofitted to existing dental unit suction equipment or alternatively fitted to central suction unit serving multiple surgeries. If *all* waste pipes carrying waste amalgam discharge from individual surgeries via the same waste water pipeline then a separator can be installed on the ultimate outflow pipe from the premises. Safe removal of the waste mercury and disposal of the separated material is the final stage of the process. The dentist is responsible for ensuring that the mercury waste is collected and treated by a waste contractor whose facilities are licenced for the recovery and disposal of hazardous amalgam waste.

A mercury spillage kit (see Box 10.3) should be kept readily available for use in the event of an accident. Never use a vacuum cleaner or suction apparatus to clear up a mercury/amalgam spillage as this will vaporise the mercury causing toxic fumes to be vented into the surgery.

Box 10.3 Mercury spillage kit

- Bulb aspirator for the collection of large drops of mercury
- White-lidded leakproof receptacle fitted with a seal and mercury suppressant (absorbent paste made of equal parts of calcium hydroxide, flowers of sulphur and water)
- Vapour mask
- Disposable gloves
- Paper towels
- Conduct a risk assessment for mercury spillages, draw up a local policy for handling spillages and train staff accordingly

---

HEALTH CARE WASTE MANAGEMENT

SEGREGATION AND DISPOSAL OF CLINICAL WASTE

Best practice guide: segregation of waste

- Segregation
  - Stage 1: Separate hazardous (clinical) waste from non-hazardous (trade and domestic waste) streams
  - Stage 2: Separate health care wastes for incineration (medicine and anatomical waste) from wastes that can be disposed of by alternative technology treatment (infectious clinical waste)
- Use nationally accepted colour-coded waste sacks and sharps bins to distinguish between different types of waste streams (see Table 10.2)
- Never use waste sacks to dispose of sharps (i.e. any item that could potentially puncture the bag) or liquids; these should be disposed of in puncture and leakproof receptacles
- Dispose of non-hazardous trade and domestic waste in black (or clear) plastic waste bag (e.g. paper, packaging, food, paper towels used for drying hands). Segregate for recycling according to local council by-laws
- Return clinical waste generated during domiciliary visits back to the practice in a suitable waste container for disposal
- Dispose of hazardous clinical waste (not sharps or medicines) into appropriately labelled UN-type leak and tear-resistant orange yellow waste sacks
- Dispose of anatomical waste for incineration in a yellow waste sack
- Suspend waste sacks in a foot-operated pedal bin. Each clinical area should have ready access to at least one orange/yellow sacks pedal bin
- Discard waste sacks when three-quarters full, and securely tie, label and date with name of practice and premises code prior to disposal (Figure 10.5 shows the swan neck method of securing the waste bag.)
- Keep manual handling of waste sacks and receptacles to a minimum. Ensure that waste containers are kept upright during use or when full
- Do not transfer waste items between clinical waste sacks

Procedures for disposal of sharps and medicines waste

- Hazardous infectious sharps must be disposed of in orange (or yellow depending on local arrangements)-lidded rigid puncture-proof containers that

HEALTH CARE WASTE MANAGEMENT

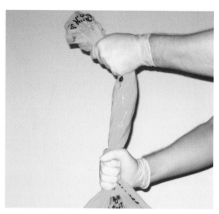
Step 1

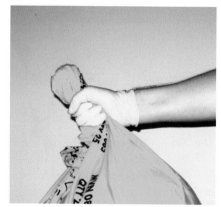
Step 2

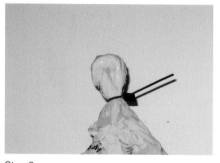
Step 3

Figure 10.5 Steps in making a 'swan neck' tie to close a hazardous waste sack. (Photograph kindly supplied by Dr Geoff Scott, Infection Control Services Ltd.)

conform to UN3291 (British Standard 7320:1990). Dispose of containers and seal when three-fourths full. Keep away from direct sources of heat. Label with the premises code and the EWC code (e.g. 18 01 03)

- Some waste contractors may be able to accept and process mixed waste containing a combination of infectious sharps waste and non-hazardous medicines sharps waste, e.g. fully discharged local anaesthetic cartridges and needles; state on the documentations that the waste is mixed and give both codes, e.g. 18 01 03 and 18 01 09

- It is not considered acceptable practice to intentionally discharge syringes containing residual local anaesthetic solution into the sink with the intention of then disposing of them into the 'fully discharged' sharps receptacle

- Medicines waste including partially discharged local anaesthetic cartridges must be segregated from other sharps waste or clinical waste and disposed of in yellow-lidded puncture-proof bins and sent for incineration (EWC code 18 01 09)

SAFE HANDLING AND STORAGE OF CLINICAL AND HAZARDOUS WASTE PRIOR TO DISPOSAL

If those handling waste are suitably trained in the segregation and disposal of waste then according to the WHO the actual risk of infection from health care waste should be minimal, accepting of course needle-stick and other sharps injuries. Therefore, as a precautionary measure any person who handles waste in the dental practice must be immunised against hepatitis B (including cleaning staff). During disposal of clinical waste, health care personnels should don the appropriate personal protective equipment (e.g. heavy duty gloves and plastic apron) to protect themselves and their clothes against spills and sharps. Hand hygiene should be performed after handling waste. If there is a risk from exposure to aerosols and splatter then masks and protective eyewear should be worn (see Chapter 6).

In the event of a sharps injury or splashing follow the guidance described in Chapter 4. Record the incident on an accident report form and assess what went wrong in order to prevent similar occurrences from happening again. Incidents often relate to breaches in the policy on handling, transportation or disposal of waste:

- Build-up of waste in an inappropriate site

- Pest control issues

- Sharps extruding from overfilled waste bins

- Sharps inadvertently placed in waste sacks

Waste carts are often heavily contaminated with pathogenic bacteria. So, care should always be taken to prevent the escape or leakage from waste sacks or containers. It is good practice to keep a body fluid spillage kit in a convenient place close to where waste for collection is stored (see Chapter 8), so that incidents can be dealt with promptly.

Best practice guide: storage of waste

- Waste should be stored in a dedicated area prior to collection

- Clinical waste sacks and bins awaiting collection should be stored in a UN-type rigid locked waste cart with a well-fitting lid

- Waste storage area should be clean, secure, well lit and inaccessible to unauthorised persons or pests

- Waste should be stored on an impervious hard surface that can be washed down should there be a spillage

HEALTH CARE WASTE MANAGEMENT

- Waste should be collected at frequent intervals to prevent a build-up of waste sacks. The actual frequency will be dictated by the volume of waste generated

TRANSPORT OF CLINICAL WASTE

Completing consignment notes for hazardous waste and keeping records

Every movement of hazardous waste (technically referred to as consigning) must be accompanied by a completed multi-part consignment note. This must be signed at each stage during the transfer of waste from the practice to the waste disposal site. This ensures 'cradle to grave' tracking of the movement of waste.

Best practice guide: consignment notes for hazardous waste

- The dentist (consignor) before collection and removal of the waste must complete the annex of the consignment note (containing a written description of the waste with the appropriate EWC code) and both the carrier and the dentist (consignor) must sign the note

- Consignment note includes the following information to prevent subsequent mismanagement of the waste:

  - The EWC code

  - A written description of the waste

  - Information about the hazardous nature of the waste and if applicable each hazardous substance

  - The weight of the waste to be consigned

  - Number of waste containers and their colour and size

- The carrier must then give a copy to both the waste producer (dentist) and the waste disposal contractor (consignee)

- The waste disposal contractor will send returns (evidence that their waste has been treated and disposed of correctly) to the dentist usually in the form of a copy consignment note. The waste contractor will also have a duty to notify the Environment Agency of the amount of hazardous waste collected, treated or disposed of and they will be charged by the agency accordingly. They are likely to pass on this charge to the producer (dental practice)

- Practices are required to keep records of the hazardous waste they produce

HEALTH CARE WASTE MANAGEMENT

- Transfer notes are to be kept for 2 years
- Consignment notes plus the return from the consignee certifying receipt of the waste for a period of 3 years from the date the waste was removed

The stated aim of the national waste strategy is to reduce the amount of health care waste produced each year. So, not surprisingly the regulations are drafted in such a way as to actively encourage practices to evaluate their activities and explore methods to limit waste generation and curb pollution. Cost savings can be made by both correct segregation of clinical waste and recycling of non-clinical waste, for example, stopping unnecessary incineration of waste that can be treated effectively with low-temperature alternative technology processes. Incineration not only contributes to global warming but also is up to ten times more expensive than low-temperature processing. Penalties are imposed on those dental practices that fail to dispose of waste in the correct manner. Dentists are liable to fines and prosecution by HSE, Environment Agency and investigation before the General Dental Council for misconduct and failure of a duty of care.

REFERENCES AND WEBSITES

Department of Health (2006). Environment and sustainability health technical Memorandum 07-01. In: *Safe Management of Healthcare Waste*. Available at http://www.dh.gov.uk.

FURTHER READING

BDA Advice note 76. Healthcare waste management. Revised November 2007. Available at http://www.bda.org.uk.

HEALTH CARE WASTE MANAGEMENT

Chapter 11

Transport and postage of diagnostic specimens, impressions and equipment for servicing and repair

LEGAL FRAMEWORK

The transport of infectious items sent by post or courier (e.g. diagnostic clinical specimens, impressions or dental equipment requiring servicing and repair) is governed by the national and international regulations on the Carriage of Dangerous Goods by Road (ADR). These regulations are intended to prevent accidental exposure of people, vehicles or machinery to hazardous materials whilst a package is in transit. In this era of heightened awareness of bioterrorism, correct and safe packaging of infectious items has taken on renewed importance. Compliance with the regulations by the health care community is essential if airlines and courier services are to continue transporting clinical material.

Note that these regulations are based on the United Nations Model Regulations for the Transport of Dangerous Goods, which are revised every 2 years (www.who.int/csr/resources/publications/biosafety). The United Nations (UN) recently altered its method for classifying pathogens for the purposes of international transport. Pathogens will no longer be assigned according to their ACDP Hazard Group; instead they are divided into two new categories, A and B (see Table 11.1). Some substances, however, are not subject to this classification and the exemptions relevant to dentistry are outlined below.

COLLECTING SPECIMENS

The regulations define clinical specimens as any substance, tissue or liquid, removed from the patients for the purpose of analysis. Specimens must be placed in leakproof container immediately after collection, either dry or in transport media, and the lid securely fastened. The patient's details must be entered on both the outside of the container and the request form. Then the container is

Table 11.1 UN categories for the transport of infectious substances

Category	Definition	UN number	Proper shipping name
A	'An infectious substance which is transported in a form that, when exposure to it occurs, is capable of causing permanent disability, life-threatening or fatal disease in otherwise healthy humans or animals' (*Based on the professional judgement known medical history and symptoms of the patient or endemic local conditions*)	UN 2814	Infectious substance affecting humans
B	'An infectious substance which does not meet the criteria for inclusion in Category A'	UN 3373	BIOLOGICAL SUBSTANCE, CATEGORY B

Modified from the World Health Organization (WHO). Guidance on Regulations for the Transport of Infectious Substances 2005.

placed in a plastic transport bag and the accompanying request form is kept into a separate pouch to avoid contamination.

Best practice guide: reducing the risk of cross-infection or injury when handling specimens

- Only staff trained to do so should handle specimens

- Specimen container should be placed in the bag separately from the request form and then placed in the designated carrying box. Staples, pins or paper clips should not be used to seal or attach forms to the bag

- Leaking and broken specimen containers should be disposed of as hazardous waste and any spillage cleaned up promptly

- Masks, protective eyewear and gloves should be worn when taking specimens

- Hands should be thoroughly cleaned after handling specimens

- Specimens should not be placed in areas where food is eaten or stored (e.g. kitchen fridge)

TRANSPORT OF SPECIMENS TO THE LABORATORY

Sending non-fixed diagnostic specimens by post

ADR classifications

According to the ADR (2007) classifications, clinical specimens taken from dental patients for diagnostic purposes are assigned to UN 3373 category B infectious substances (diagnostic or clinical specimens). Clinical samples from dental practices transferred to hospital or private laboratories should be packed according to ADR Packing Instructions P650 for road transport or the IATA packing instruction 650 for air transport. These packaging instructions are based on the use of the UN triple-package system (Figure 11.1) which is commercially available from suppliers. Home-made packaging is to be avoided as this is unlikely to be compliant. Packaging for category B infectious substances must be capable of passing a 1.2-m drop test. This means that following a drop from a height of 1.2 m, there is no leakage from the primary receptacle and this should remain protected by the absorbent material within the secondary packaging.

The World Health Organization (WHO) recommends a basic triple-packaging system which is suitable for all infectious substances. It consists of three layers.

Labelling

Each completed package is required to be marked, labelled and accompanied with appropriate shipping documents (as applicable). Outer packaging is labelled with the proper shipping name in letters at least 6 mm high, i.e. 'BIOLOGICAL SUBSTANCE CATEGORY B' and display the symbol shown in Figure 11.2. Copies of the paper work should also be enclosed within the packaging plus an emergency response procedure in case of accidents. For airfreight,

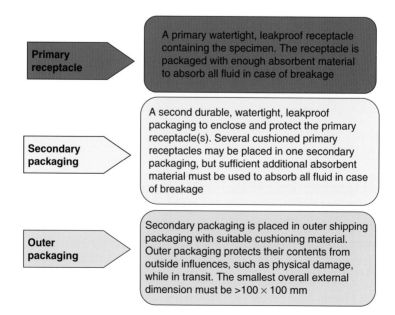

Primary receptacle — A primary watertight, leakproof receptacle containing the specimen. The receptacle is packaged with enough absorbent material to absorb all fluid in case of breakage

Secondary packaging — A second durable, watertight, leakproof packaging to enclose and protect the primary receptacle(s). Several cushioned primary receptacles may be placed in one secondary packaging, but sufficient additional absorbent material must be used to absorb all fluid in case of breakage

Outer packaging — Secondary packaging is placed in outer shipping packaging with suitable cushioning material. Outer packaging protects their contents from outside influences, such as physical damage, while in transit. The smallest overall external dimension must be >100 × 100 mm

Figure 11.1 WHO triple packaging.

Figure 11.2 UN biological substance category B symbol.

complete an airway bill form that is supplied by the airline. Packages should be clearly labelled with the delivery address and sender's details with emergency contact details including a named person, at both where the package is being sent from and where it is going to, and a telephone number in case of leaks or queries.

Packages containing liquids must show package orientation labels. Failure to comply with the postal and transport packaging regulations may lead to prosecution.

TRANSPORT RESTRICTIONS

Public transport

Category B infectious substances must not be carried by a member of staff on their person or in a bag on public transport. Similarly, infectious substances in category A or category B are not permitted for transport in carry-on or checked baggage on airlines, nor may they be carried on the person. A member of staff transporting clinical samples as part of their work would be expected to comply with the ADR regulations, whereas, a dental patient is permitted to take their clinical sample to a dental surgery on public transport, as this is outside the remit of the ADR regulations.

Mail and courier services

Royal mail will accept category B diagnostic specimens provided they are packaged to P650 requirements. For transport by road (private car or courier service), there are no limits on the quantity of materials allowed within either the primary receptacle(s) or the total package. This is in contrast to air transport either by passenger or by cargo aircraft where other than for body parts (or whole bodies) there is a 4 L/4 kg limit per package, with a 1-L limit per primary receptacle for liquids, whereas for solids, the primary receptacle must not exceed the outer packaging mass limit of 4 kg (International Air Transport Association (IATA); http://www.iataonline.com).

TRANSPORT AND POSTAGE OF
DIAGNOSTIC SPECIMENS

FIXED PATHOLOGICAL SPECIMENS

Several types of clinical diagnostic specimens are exempted from the ADR regulations:

- Blood specimens for biochemical tests, e.g. blood glucose levels where it is assumed that such specimens would be free of pathogens unless the patient is a carrier of a blood-borne virus infection

- Fixed histopathology specimens: pathogens that might have been present in the specimen are destroyed by the fixation process

Both types of specimens are not considered to be a health risk unless they meet the criteria for inclusion in another class, e.g. contain toxic or radioactive chemicals. A condition of eligibility for the exemption criteria requires that the specimens are appropriately packaged for posting and shipping.

Packaging

Oral pathological specimens for histopathology are placed in a leakproof container filled with formalin with a screw-top cap and placed in a self-sealing plastic bag. The pathology request form which identifies the specimen must be placed in a separate plastic bag from the specimen. If the specimen container leaks then the patient's information is not contaminated and remains legible.

The packaging must comply with the following ADR requirements to prevent any leakage occurring. The packaging consists of three components:

1. A leakproof primary receptacle(s)

2. A leakproof secondary packaging

3. Outer packaging of adequate strength for its capacity, mass and intended use, and with at least one surface having minimum dimensions of 100 × 100 mm

When sending several specimens in the same packaging then individually wrap tubes/bottles or use a box with dividers to avoid breakages occurring in transit. For liquid specimens, place sufficient absorbent material between the primary receptacle(s) and the secondary packaging both to cushion the specimen from breakage and to absorb the entire volume of liquid in case of a leak. This will prevent compromising the integrity of the outer packaging and avoid contaminating persons handling the package or sorting office machinery. The outer padded leakproof postal packet should be clearly marked with the words

'Exempt human specimen' and the name and address of the sender (and person to be contacted in case of leakage or queries) and that of the recipient.

TRANSPORTING IMPRESSIONS

In response to the commercial advantages of the 'global market place', it is not uncommon for dentists to send dental impression to laboratories overseas. Regardless of whether the impressions are sent to a laboratory in the UK or overseas, the transport and postal regulations will apply. However, if the impression is thoroughly disinfected as described in Chapter 7, then it will no longer pose an infection hazard, making it exempt under the ADR regulations for category B substances. The packaging requirements described for fixed diagnostic specimens will still apply. Packaging can be reused unless it becomes soiled or damaged.

EQUIPMENT TO BE SENT FOR SERVICE OR REPAIR

Dental equipment, which has been contaminated with blood/body fluids or has been exposed to patients with a known infectious disease, should be decontaminated before being dispatched to third parties for service or repair. The same principles apply as for diagnostic specimens, namely that the device or equipment should not expose the recipient to biological, chemical or radiation hazards. In some circumstances, it may be necessary to seek additional advice from the manufacturer on the most appropriate mode of decontamination, especially for electronic or electrical equipment. Accompanying the equipment should be a written declaration providing the following information on the contamination status:

- It is contaminated with blood, body fluids, pathogens or hazardous chemicals
- It has been cleaned and/or decontaminated
- The method used for cleaning, disinfection or sterilization
- Signed and dated to declare that 'the item has been prepared to ensure safe handling and transportation'

(Forms can be obtained from Medicines and Healthcare Products Agency website at http://devices.mhra.gov.uk.)

If it is not possible to decontaminate the equipment (e.g. if it requires dismantling by engineer in order to be able to clean the interior), then the repair

TRANSPORT AND POSTAGE OF
DIAGNOSTIC SPECIMENS

company should be contacted and asked if they will accept a contaminated item. When dispatching devices via mail or courier, the shipping and packaging requirements described above will apply. If the repair company does not agree to the dispatch of the device, then quarantine the item, label with its contamination status and arrange a site visit to the practice by the company.

FURTHER READING

Department of Health (2005). *Changes to the Infectious Substances Transport Procedures in 2005*. England, UK: Department of Health. Available at http//www.dh.gov.uk/publications.

Department of Health (June 2007). *Transport of Infectious Substances – Best Practice Guidance for Microbiology Laboratories*. England, UK: Inspector of Microbiology and Infection Control, Department of Health. Available at http://www.dh.gov.uk/publications.

TRANSPORT AND POSTAGE OF DIAGNOSTIC SPECIMENS

Chapter 12
Appendix

Table 12.1 Daily infection control clinical pathway

At start of the day

- Remove watch and rings (except wedding rings). Work bare below the elbows; wash hands with plain or medicated soap
- Fill the steriliser reservoir with reverse osmosis (RO) or sterile water
- Confirm the steriliser is working correctly by completing an automatic control test (for all types of sterilisers) and steam penetration test (for vacuum sterilisers)
- Store printout or record the cycle sterilisation parameters (temperature, pressure and holding time) in sterilizer logbook; record if passed or failed tests
- Check sufficient sterile instruments are available for the session. Run steriliser as required; record cycle number in patient's notes
- Don heavy duty gloves, apron and goggles for cleaning surfaces with disinfectant and preparing fresh solutions of detergents and disinfectants
- Fill dental unit waterlines reservoir with RO, distilled or sterile water. Flush lines for 2 minutes. Replenish biocide in waterlines
- Prepare fresh solution of detergent for ultrasonic bath, fill with solution and run bath empty for 2 minutes to degas bath; function test regularly
- Check all clinical surfaces are clean and free of clutter. Wipe all surfaces with a hard surface cleaner. Clean chair and headrest
- Switch on air conditioning or open windows to ensure good ventilation

In preparation for patient treatment

- Cover chair, light switches, handles, suction and air and waterlines with disposable coverings. Items can be passed into 'dirty zones' but contaminated items should not be passed out into 'clean zones'
- Place sterile instrument set on the bracket table and lay out all materials to be used in the clean zone. Storage containers of dental materials should not be placed in the 'dirty zone'

During patient treatment

- Recheck patient's medical history. Patient's notes, radiographs and computers should remain in the clean zone and not be touched with gloved hands
- Observe standard precautions; treat all patients as potentially infectious
- Place goggles and bib on the patient
- Clean hands with alcohol hand rub before and after removing gloves at the end of procedure

(Continued)

Table 12.1 (*Continued*)

- Don personal protective equipment (PPE) (gloves, masks, protective eyewear and clothing). Change between patients and dispose of as clinical waste (yellow or orange waste sack)
- Reduce aerosols contamination by the use of high-volume suction and rubber dam (if appropriate)
- Work sharp safe: use resheathing device or safety syringes or single-handed technique to dispose of needles
- Clinician should dispose of single-use sharps (needles, sutures, scalpels, steel burs) and fully discharged Local Anaesthetic cartridges into clinical (hazardous) waste 'sharps bin' immediately after use. Only fill to three-fourths full
- Segregate medicines waste, e.g. partially discharged LA cartridges and needles from other sharps waste (yellow-lidded sharps bin for incineration)
- Dispose of amalgam waste in a special white-lidded mercury waste receptacle
- Remove disposable coverings at the end of treatment and dispose of as clinical waste

After treatment (wear appropriate PPE, remove before leaving treatment or decontamination area; clean hands before and after removing gloves)

- **In treatment room**: Clean and disinfect all contaminated work surfaces in the dirty zone
- Rinse and disinfect impressions and other dental appliances before sending to laboratory
- Prepare surgery for next patient; flush waterlines for 30 seconds between patients
- **Instrument decontamination**: Transport instruments to decontamination room/area in clean container with secure lid. Deposit in dirty zone
- Strictly segregate dirty from clean instruments
- Clean hands and don fresh PPE, e.g. apron, heavy duty gloves (protective eyewear and mask if manually cleaning instruments)
- Pre-soak instruments if cannot be cleaned immediately
- Whenever possible keep instruments together in their trays, for instrument tracking
- Clean instruments in ultrasonic bath (metal instruments only) or preferably use washer disinfector fitted with connectors for handpieces, dry and inspect to ensure visibly clean. Wrap instruments if using a vacuum sterilizer
- Disinfect and lubricate handpieces (preferably in an automated handpiece cleaner)
- Sterilize instruments at 134°C for 3 minutes; keep cycle printout
- Store dry instruments in covered trays or instrument packs in clean dry environment; use stock control
- Remove PPE and clean hands with alcohol hand rub or soap and water on exiting the room

At the end of each session, clean hands before and after removing gloves

- Clean and disinfect all work surfaces thoroughly in both dirty and clean zones
- Wipe down the dental chair, bracket table, tubing and spittoon
- Drain off water in sterilizer and replace with freshly prepared or bottled water
- Do not eat or store food or drink in the treatment or decontamination room

At the end of the day, clean hands before and after removing gloves

- Dispose of all clinical waste sacks from treatment room and store in secure area
- Disinfect the aspirator, its tubing and the spittoon, and clean trap

Table 12.1 (*Continued*)

- Drain down dental unit waterline and disinfect (if not using a continuous dosing systems). Empty and disinfect reservoir bottle. Store dry and inverted
- Drain down and clean ultrasonic bath, and leave dry
- Clean steriliser chamber and inspect seals
- Empty and drain sterilizer water reservoir; clean and leave dry
- Dispose of any partially used bottles of water as they will be contaminated
- Change out of tunic/uniform and launder daily

Note: This is an outline only; read best practice guides for more detailed protocols.

Table 12.2 Decontamination methods for specific instruments and items of dental equipment

Item	Decontamination requirements
Airways and endotracheal tubes	Single-use items. Any reusable items should be steam sterilized
Bracket table and handle	Cover with cling film during use; then disinfect with surface disinfectant, e.g. alcohol wipe
Brushes (for cleaning equipment)	Discard, or clean and autoclave following use. Store dry
Burs (diamond, tungsten carbide)	Immerse in enzymic disinfectant; follow manufacturer's instructions on dilution and immersion time. Steam sterilise and dry
Burs (steel)	Steel burs are a single-use item
Carpets	Not suitable for clinical areas
	Vacuum regularly (normally daily). Steam clean periodically
Curing light	Cover tip with cling film or impervious plastic sleeve. (Tips also available as sterilizer or as single-use disposable.) Wipe outer casing with surface disinfectant or alcohol wipe after use on each patient
Dappens pot	Glass: clean and steam steriliser; plastic: single-use disposable
Dental chair and stools	Covering should be intact. Clean regularly with warm water and detergent. Blood/body fluid splashes should be cleaned immediately with *dilute* hypochlorite solution and wiped with a manufacturer-recommended surface disinfectant
Dental chair switches	Cover with cling film; change between patients; end of session disinfect with surface disinfectant
Dental handpieces and connectors	Automatic cleaning device recommended or cleaning and pre-oiling according to handpiece manufacturer's instructions prior to placement in vacuum (or if not available a non-vacuum) sterilizer. Handpiece couplings and hose cover with impervious sleeve/cling film; clean with surface disinfectant
Endodontic instruments	Endodontic files and reamers are single use only

(Continued)

Table 12.2 (*Continued*)

Item	Decontamination requirements
	If designated reusable by manufacturer, e.g. some rotary files, then brush clean, soak in an enzymic cleaner, and place in ultrasonic bath and steam sterilise. Bent or damaged instrument should be discarded
Extracted teeth to be used for educational purposes	Remove amalgam restorations from the teeth and dispose into special amalgam hazardous waste receptacle, labelled as 18 01 10. Disinfect teeth for 10 minutes in freshly prepared 1:10 dilution of hypochlorite, rinse in sterile water, dry and then store in a leakproof container immersed in a second freshly prepared 1:10 solution of hypochlorite
Face bows	Remove debris and clean with surface disinfectant; steam sterilise the fork
Fan (mechanical) and air conditioning	Avoid use of fans in clinical areas as difficult to clean effectively. If use is considered essential, then routinely wipe clean with detergent. Regularly change filters and clean air-conditioning units
Furniture and fittings	Should be in good repair and all coverings intact. Damp dust with warm water and detergent. If known contamination, wash with diluted hypochlorite solution. Choose furniture upholstered with wipeable fabrics
Forceps	Manual cleaning and ultrasonic bath or thermal washer disinfector; steam sterilise; store in clean dry container/tray. Preferably sterilised in pouches in a vacuum steriliser
Kidney dishes	Manual cleaning or thermal washer disinfector, steam sterilizer; or single-use disposables
Light handles	Cover with cling film/impermeable cover and replace between patients. Clean with surface disinfectant at end of session
Masks	Single-use disposable
Matrix bands	Single-use disposable
Metal syringes	Automated cleaning in a thermal washer disinfector or manually cleaning followed by steam sterilisation. Plastic syringes are single-use only
Nail brushes	Single-use only (generally not recommended for hand hygiene in dental practice)
Needles	Single-use item. Resheath carefully with finger guard protectors or other resheathing device or if not available single-handed scoop method. Dispose of plastic syringes and needles as one unit into sharps bin. Consider using retractable safety needles
Plastic aprons	Single use
Paper points	Use pre-sterilized packs
Radiographic film	Handle with gloves; use barrier pouch
Radiographic film holders and positioning devices	Sterilize; if not heat tolerant then clean by immersion in disinfectant
Radiograph tube – heads and control panels	Protect with cling film (impervious barrier); change after each patient

Table 12.2 (*Continued*)

Item	Decontamination requirements
Spittoon	Clean outer surface first. Inner surface of bowl – add (metered) dose of non-foaming disinfectant, wipe evenly around inside of bowl, leave for time interval specified by manufacturer, rinse with bowl flush and then discard disinfection cloth
Stethoscopes	Use 70% isopropyl alcohol wipes on bell and earpieces
Suction tips	If reusable then clean manually (metal tips can be cleaned in an ultrasonic bath), or in thermal washer disinfector, steam sterilise
	Disposable suction tips, single-use only
Suction lines	Trap filters must be removed and cleaned every night with a non-foaming disinfectant and rinsed thoroughly before replacing. Do not use bleach or hypochlorite with a metal filter as it causes rusting. Tubing and lines disinfected with a non-foaming disinfectant/detergent and left overnight as specified in manufacturer's instructions
Thermometer	High-level disinfection according to manufacturer's instructions or use disposable strips. DO NOT AUTOCLAVE as contains mercury
Ultrasonic scalers and handle	Scalers are steam sterilised, cover handles in cling film or impervious plastic sleeves that are changed after each use and wipe connector and hose with surface disinfectant

Note: The list is not exhaustive.

Table 12.3 Hand and hard-surface disinfectants and dental unit waterline biocides

Type of disinfectant/antiseptic	Proprietary name	Use in dental surgery
Chlorhexidines		
Chlorhexidine gluconate liquid 4%	Hibiscrub surgical scrub	Hand washing
Chlorhexidine 2.5% in 70% alcohol solution in a glycerine base	Hibisol handrub	Hand rub
Chlorhexidine 0.5% in 70% alcohol	Alcoholic chlorhexidine	Skin disinfection prior to perioral biopsy, implant surgery and periodontal surgery
Chlorhexidine gluconate 0.12% and ethanol 12%	Bio Blue	Biocide for disinfection for dental unit waterlines and reservoir bottles
Iodophors		
Povidone iodine 7.5% solution	Betadine surgical scrub	Hand washing

(*Continued*)

APPENDIX

Table 12.3 (*Continued*)

Type of disinfectant/antiseptic	Proprietary name	Use in dental surgery
Alcohols		
Alcohol gel/solutions	Purell, Sterillium, Desderman	Hand rub
70% Isopropyl alcohol wipes	Azowipes or cliniwipes	Surgery hard-surface disinfection or external surface of handpieces
Ethanol and 1-propanol alcohol spray	Mikrozoid	Surgery hard-surface disinfection
Chlorine-releasing agents		
Sodium dichloroisocyanurate solution tablets 4.75 g (=2.5 g available chlorine) or granules	Haz-tabs tablet or granules	Spillage of blood or other body fluids
	Presept tablets or granules	
Sodium hypochlorite + detergent	Chloros	Surgery hard-surface disinfection
Chlorine dioxide	Tristel (chlorine dioxide-releasing wipes	Surgery hard-surface disinfection
Triclosan		
Triclosan 2%	Aquasept	Hand disinfection
Phenolic		
Hycolin 2% solution	Stericol	Disinfection of environmental surfaces, e.g. floors
Halogenic alkyl + aryl phenolic	Orotol	Suction tubing disinfectant
Peracetic acid		
Peracetic acid	Nu-cidex	High-level disinfection of heat-labile instruments, *only* for intermediate and low-risk procedures
	Gigasept PA	
Superoxidised water		
Electrolysed salt solution produced by a dedicated generator (releases oxidising agents and chlorine)	Sterilox	Biocide for disinfection of dental unit waterlines and reservoir bottles
Alkaline peroxide based		
Alkaline peroxide	Sterilex ultra	Biocide for disinfection of dental unit waterlines and reservoir bottles
Hydrogen peroxide, silver ions	Dentisept P, Oxygenal 6, Sanosil Super 25	
Citric acid based		
Sodium hypochlorite, citric acid	Alpron	Biocide for disinfection of dental unit waterlines and reservoir bottles

Note: The list contains examples only and is not exhaustive.

APPENDIX

FURTHER SOURCES OF INFORMATION

- **Medicines and Healthcare Products Regulatory Agency (MHRA)**

  http://www.mhra.gov.uk

  List of all current device bulletins on sterilisers/sterilising instruments and product safety warnings

- **Department of Health and the Department of Health Estates and Facilities Directorate**

  Hosted by the Department of Health website

  http://www.dh.gov.uk

  Excellent source of technical information on decontamination and latest regulations relating to infection control

- **Environment Agency**

  http://www.environment-agency.gov.uk

  Information on waste disposal and notification of waste producer premises

- **Health and Safety Executive**

  http://www.hse.gov.uk

  For health and safety information and RIDDOR (Reporting of Injuries, Diseases and Dangerous Occurrences) forms

- **Health Protection Agency**

  http://www.hpa.org.uk

  Information on infection control and related infection and health topics, disease outbreaks, and national and regional health statistics and surveillance data

- **World Health Organization**

  http://www.who.int/

  Information on infection control and related topics, disease outbreaks, and international health statistics

- **ICS Ltd.**

  http://www.infectioncontrolservices.co.uk

  Web-based infection control manual

APPENDIX

- **British Dental Association**

  http://www.bda.org

  National professional association for dentists. Downloadable infection control manual (BDA Advice Sheet A12), waste disposal guidance and information for dentists on legal, employment and clinical governance aspects of infection control

Index